1. Introduction to Physiotherapy

- Definition of physiotherapy

- Brief history and evolution

- Importance of physiotherapy in modern medicine

- The role of physiotherapists

- Common misconceptions about physiotherapy

2. How Physiotherapy Works

- Overview of human anatomy and biomechanics

- How physiotherapy targets muscles, bones, and joints

- The science behind physiotherapy techniques

- Differences between physiotherapy and other forms of rehabilitation

3. Common Conditions Treated with Physiotherapy

- Musculoskeletal conditions

- Neurological conditions

- Cardiopulmonary issues

- Pediatric physiotherapy

- Geriatric physiotherapy for elderly individuals

4. Benefits of Physiotherapy for General Population

- Improved mobility and flexibility

- Pain management without medication

- Injury prevention

- Better posture and body mechanics

- Mental health benefits

5. Physiotherapy for Common Injuries

- Sports injuries

- Work-related injuries

- Post-operative rehabilitation

 - ACL reconstruction

- Hip/knee replacement

- Fracture recovery and physiotherapy's role

- Shoulder injuries

6. Physiotherapy Techniques and Modalities

- Manual therapy techniques

- Therapeutic exercises and stretches

- Electrotherapy

- Hydrotherapy

- Dry needling and acupuncture in physiotherapy

- Use of heat and cold therapy

7. Home Exercises and Self-Care

- Basic stretching routines for different body parts

- Core strengthening exercises for stability

- Exercises for posture correction

- Injury prevention strategies through exercise

- Guidelines on ergonomics and correct posture at home and work

8. Physiotherapy for Special Populations

- Physiotherapy during pregnancy

- Physiotherapy for children with developmental disorders

- Geriatric care and fall prevention

- Physiotherapy for athletes

- Working with patients with chronic pain

9. Case Studies

- Case study 1: Physiotherapy for chronic back pain

- Case study 2: Stroke recovery with physiotherapy

- Case study 3: Post-operative rehabilitation for joint replacement

- Case study 4: Sports injury recovery using physiotherapy

- Case study 5: Pediatric physiotherapy success story

10. Future of Physiotherapy

- Advancements in technology

- Integration of AI in physiotherapy treatments

- Innovations in rehabilitation techniques

- Global trends in physiotherapy education and practice

11. How to Choose the Right Physiotherapist

- Qualifications and certifications to look for

- Questions to ask during the consultation

- Red flags to avoid

- Understanding the treatment plan and setting realistic goals

12. Frequently Asked Questions (FAQ) About Physiotherapy

- What can I expect during my first physiotherapy session?

- How long do physiotherapy sessions typically last?

- How many sessions do I need?

- Is physiotherapy painful?

- Can physiotherapy help with chronic conditions?

13. Overview of Physiotherapy

- Assessment and Diagnosis

- Treatment Techniques

- Conditions Treated

- Goals of Physiotherapy

1. Introduction to Physiotherapy:-

A) Definition of physiotherapy:-

 Physiotherapy, also known as physical therapy, is a healthcare profession that focuses on diagnosing, treating, and preventing physical impairments, disabilities, and pain. It uses various physical methods like exercises, manual therapy, movement training, and electrotherapy to restore mobility, improve strength, and enhance functional ability. Physiotherapists work to rehabilitate patients with musculoskeletal, neurological, and cardiopulmonary conditions, among others, aiming to improve their quality of life and independence.

B) Brief history and evolution:-

Physiotherapy has a rich history that dates back to ancient times. Its roots can be traced to the early practices of manual therapy and therapeutic exercises, used by civilizations like the Greeks, Egyptians, and Chinese. Hippocrates, the "father of medicine," advocated massage and hydrotherapy around 460 B.C., marking one of the earliest formal approaches to physical treatment.

Key milestones in the evolution of physiotherapy:

1) 19th Century Beginnings:-
Modern physiotherapy emerged in the 19th century, influenced by advancements in orthopedic surgery and the development of massage therapy, movement techniques, and electrotherapy. Swedish gymnast Per Henrik Ling is credited with founding physical education and the development of the Swedish Movement Cure, a precursor to modern physiotherapy.

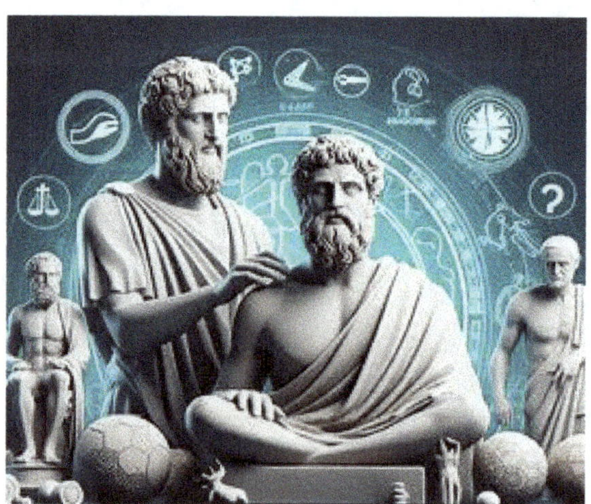

2) World War I and II:-
Physiotherapy gained prominence during and after the World Wars when physical rehabilitation was crucial for injured soldiers. Rehabilitation centers and hospitals began to employ physiotherapists to assist in restoring mobility and function, particularly for amputees and those with nerve injuries.

3) Professionalization (20ᵗʰ Century):-

In the early 20ᵗʰ century, formal organizations were established, such as the Chartered Society of Physiotherapy in the UK (1894) and the American Physical Therapy Association (1921). During this period, physiotherapists became more integrated into healthcare teams, with education and training becoming more structured.

4) Advancements in Techniques:-

Over the decades, physiotherapy expanded to incorporate more scientific and evidence-based approaches. Techniques like manual therapy, exercise prescription, and the use of electrical modalities developed further. The profession also began specializing in fields such as sports physiotherapy, pediatric therapy, and neurological rehabilitation.

5) Technological Integration (Late 20th Century – Present):-

In recent years, physiotherapy has embraced new technologies, including robotic rehabilitation, virtual reality, and tele-rehabilitation. These innovations have allowed for more precise and individualized treatment, particularly for post-surgical rehabilitation and chronic conditions.

Today, physiotherapy is a well-established global profession, recognized for its role in promoting mobility, reducing pain, and enhancing patients' overall quality of life across various medical conditions.

C) Importance of physiotherapy in modern medicine:-

Physiotherapy plays a crucial role in modern medicine due to its focus on restoring function, reducing pain, and improving quality of life without the need for medication or invasive procedures. Its importance can be summarized in several key areas:

1. **Pain Management**

Physiotherapy offers effective, non-pharmacological treatments for managing pain. Techniques like manual therapy, therapeutic exercises, and electrotherapy help reduce discomfort, promote healing, and improve patient outcomes, especially for chronic pain conditions like arthritis, back pain, and fibromyalgia.

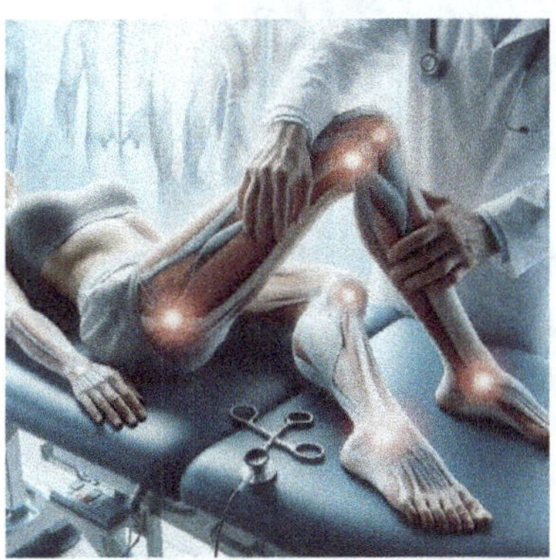

2. **Rehabilitation Post-Surgery or Injury**

Physiotherapists are essential in the recovery process after surgeries, such as joint replacements or cardiac procedures, and for injuries like fractures or sprains. They design personalized rehabilitation programs to restore movement, strength, and flexibility, speeding up recovery and preventing complications like muscle atrophy.

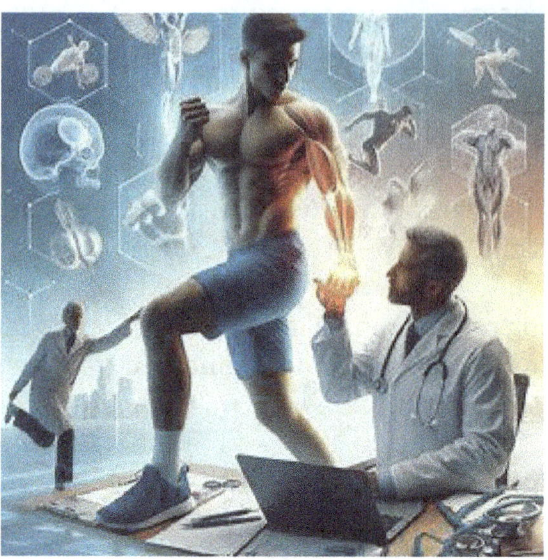

3. **Preventing Mobility Issues**

For patients with neurological conditions (such as stroke, Parkinson's disease, or multiple sclerosis), physiotherapy helps maintain and improve mobility. Early intervention can slow down the progression of these conditions, preserving independence and enhancing the quality of life.

4. **Chronic Disease Management**

Physiotherapy is valuable in managing chronic illnesses such as diabetes, heart disease, and respiratory conditions. By incorporating exercise and mobility training, physiotherapists help patients improve cardiovascular health, manage blood sugar levels, and enhance lung function, contributing to overall health.

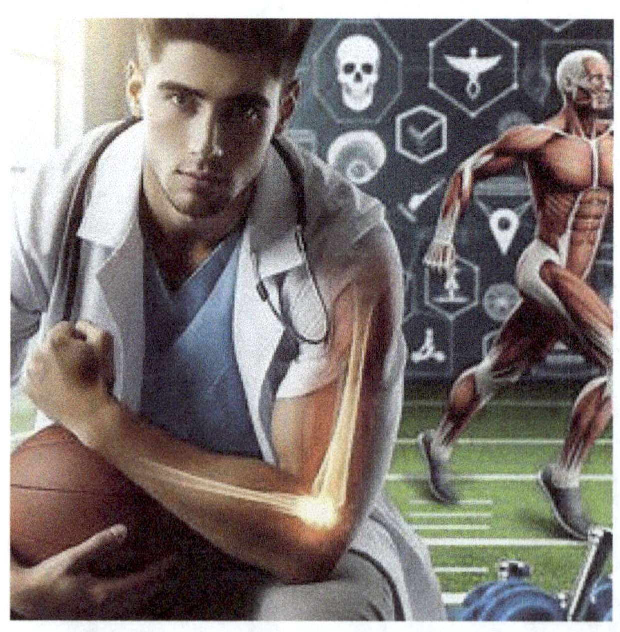

5. **Injury Prevention**

In sports and occupational settings, physiotherapy is critical for preventing injuries. It focuses on strengthening muscles, improving posture, and enhancing body mechanics, thereby reducing the risk of injuries in athletes, workers, and the elderly.

6. **Improving Quality of Life for the Elderly**

Physiotherapy plays a vital role in geriatrics by helping older adults maintain mobility, balance, and independence. It can prevent falls, treat conditions like osteoporosis, and manage age-related issues like arthritis, making it essential for enhancing the quality of life in aging populations.

7. **Non-Invasive and Cost-Effective**

As a conservative treatment, physiotherapy offers an alternative to surgeries and long-term medication use. It is often more affordable and can reduce the need for costly procedures, making it a critical component of healthcare, particularly in managing musculoskeletal and chronic conditions.

physiotherapy is integral to modern medicine for its ability to rehabilitate, prevent injuries, manage chronic conditions, and improve overall well-being, making it indispensable in healthcare systems worldwide.

D) The role of physiotherapists:-

Physiotherapists play a vital role in healthcare, specializing in the diagnosis, treatment, and prevention of movement-related disorders. Their primary aim is to help individuals restore function, improve mobility, and enhance their overall physical health. The key roles of physiotherapists include:

1. **Assessment and Diagnosis**

Physiotherapists assess patients by conducting thorough physical examinations and reviewing medical histories. They identify the root cause of physical impairments, pain, or movement restrictions and provide a diagnosis based on this evaluation.

2. **Treatment Planning**

After diagnosis, physiotherapists develop individualized treatment plans tailored to the patient's specific needs. These plans often include exercises, manual therapy, and other techniques to promote recovery, relieve pain, and improve physical function.

3. **Rehabilitation**

One of the core roles of physiotherapists is to rehabilitate patients recovering from surgery, injury, or illness. They design exercise programs and use therapeutic techniques to help patients regain strength, mobility, and coordination, facilitating their return to normal daily activities.

4. **Pain Management**

Physiotherapists employ various methods, such as manual therapy, heat/cold treatments, electrotherapy, and exercises, to help manage acute or chronic pain without the need for medication. This is particularly important in conditions like back pain, arthritis, or fibromyalgia.

5. **Preventing Injury and Disease**

DiseasePhysiotherapists work to prevent future injuries and illnesses by educating patients on proper body mechanics, posture, and ergonomics. They also design preventive exercise programs for athletes, elderly individuals, and those at risk of musculoskeletal disorders to reduce injury risks.

6. **Supporting Long-Term Health**

Physiotherapists help manage chronic conditions such as heart disease, diabetes, respiratory issues, and neurological disorders. They offer long-term support through exercise programs and lifestyle advice that help control symptoms and improve the quality of life.

7. **Collaboration with Healthcare Teams**

Physiotherapists often work as part of a multidisciplinary healthcare team, collaborating with doctors, nurses, occupational therapists, and other healthcare professionals. This ensures a holistic approach to patient care, particularly in complex cases like stroke rehabilitation or post-surgical recovery.

8. **Educating and Empowering Patients**

Physiotherapists play a key role in educating patients about their conditions and treatment options. They teach patients exercises and self-care strategies to manage their conditions independently, fostering long-term health and wellness.

9.**Specialized CareMany **

physiotherapists specialize in areas such as sports physiotherapy, pediatric therapy, geriatric care, or neurological rehabilitation. This allows them to provide more targeted care to specific populations or conditions.In summary, physiotherapists are essential for improving patients' physical well-being, promoting recovery, preventing injury, and supporting long-term health through a comprehensive and individualized approach.

E) Common misconceptions about physiotherapy:-

There are several common misconceptions about physiotherapy that often lead to misunderstandings about its scope and effectiveness. Here are a few:

1. **Physiotherapy is Only for Injuries**

Many people believe physiotherapy is only necessary after a sports injury or surgery. In reality, physiotherapists treat a wide range of conditions, including chronic diseases (e.g., arthritis, heart disease), neurological disorders (e.g., stroke, Parkinson's), respiratory issues, and postural problems.

2. **It's Just About Exercise**

While exercise is a significant component of physiotherapy, it also includes various treatments such as manual therapy, electrotherapy, ultrasound therapy, and education on body mechanics, ergonomics, and lifestyle adjustments to improve overall health and prevent injury.

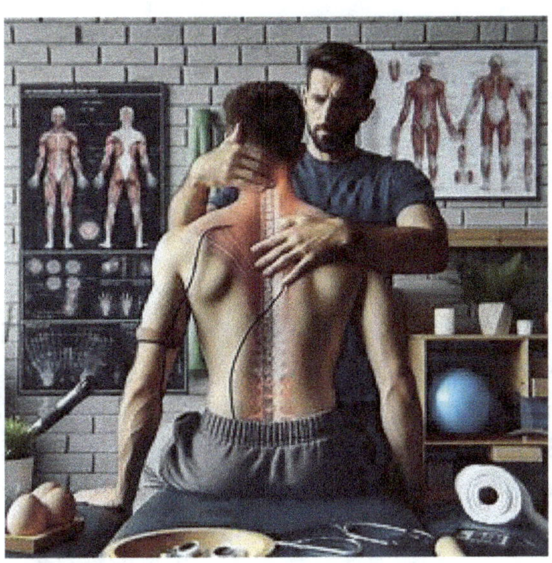

3. **Physiotherapy is Only for Athletes**

Although athletes frequently benefit from physiotherapy, it is meant for people of all ages and activity levels. Whether someone is recovering from surgery, dealing with age-related mobility issues, or managing chronic conditions, physiotherapy can be beneficial for everyone.

4. **Physiotherapy is Painful**

Many assume that physiotherapy will involve intense pain. While some discomfort may be part of rehabilitation, physiotherapists tailor treatments to the patient's tolerance and work to manage pain through gradual and controlled movements.

5. **Physiotherapy is the Same as Massage**

Though massage may be a component of physiotherapy, it is just one small aspect. Physiotherapy is a medical discipline that involves a range of evidence-based treatments, including therapeutic exercises, manual therapy, electrotherapy, and rehabilitation strategies to address specific conditions.

6. **You Need a Doctor's Referral for Physiotherapy**

In many places, physiotherapists are primary care professionals, meaning patients can seek treatment without a doctor's referral. However, in certain healthcare systems or for specific insurance purposes, a referral may still be required.

7. **Physiotherapy is Only for Rehabilitation**

Physiotherapy is not just for post-injury or post-surgery recovery. It is also widely used for preventive care, such as preventing sports injuries, managing chronic conditions, and improving overall physical health and mobility.

8. **Physiotherapy Only Focuses on Physical Problems**

While physiotherapists primarily treat physical impairments, they also address the psychological aspects of recovery. They help patients overcome fears, build confidence in movement, and manage stress, which is often linked to physical conditions like chronic pain.

These misconceptions can prevent people from seeking out the full benefits of physiotherapy, which is a highly versatile and integral part of healthcare.

2. How Physiotherapy Works:-

Physiotherapy works by assessing, diagnosing, and treating physical impairments and disabilities through movement-based exercises, manual therapy, and various therapeutic techniques. It aims to restore function, improve mobility, and reduce pain in muscles, bones, and joints. By using a combination of exercise, education, and hands-on treatment, physiotherapy helps individuals recover from injury, manage chronic conditions, and prevent future physical issues. The practice is based on principles of human anatomy, biomechanics, and the science of tissue healing.

A) Overview of human anatomy and biomechanics:-

Physiotherapy is grounded in a deep understanding of the body's structure and movement. Human anatomy involves the study of the musculoskeletal system (bones, muscles, joints, tendons, ligaments), the nervous system, and the circulatory system, among others. Biomechanics looks at how these structures work together to produce movement and maintain stability. Physiotherapists use knowledge of anatomy and biomechanics to assess movement dysfunction, identify muscle imbalances, and correct abnormal posture or gait, ensuring the body moves efficiently and painlessly.

B) How physiotherapy targets muscles, bones, and joints:-

Physiotherapy uses techniques like manual therapy, exercise prescription, and modalities (such as ultrasound and electrical stimulation) to target the muscles, bones, and joints. For muscles, physiotherapy focuses on strengthening, stretching, and restoring flexibility. It helps repair muscle tears or strains and improve muscle function. For bones, physiotherapy aids in the healing process post-fracture, or in conditions like osteoporosis. For joints, physiotherapists help restore range of motion, reduce stiffness, and relieve pain from conditions such as arthritis or joint injuries.

C) The science behind physiotherapy techniques:-

Physiotherapy techniques are based on principles of tissue healing, muscle conditioning, pain modulation, and neuroplasticity. For example, exercises promote blood flow and healing, while strengthening muscles to support bones and joints. Techniques like soft tissue mobilization or dry needling can release muscle tension and trigger healing responses. Additionally, physiotherapy embraces neuroplasticity — the brain's ability to rewire itself — to help patients regain mobility and coordination after neurological injuries like strokes or spinal cord damage.

D)Differences between physiotherapy and other forms of rehabilitation:-

While physiotherapy focuses on physical recovery through movement, strength, and flexibility, other forms of rehabilitation may involve different approaches. Occupational therapy, for example, focuses on helping people regain the ability to perform daily tasks. Speech therapy addresses communication or swallowing issues. While physiotherapy can overlap with these fields, its unique focus on biomechanics, movement patterns, and the musculoskeletal system differentiates it from other rehabilitation forms that may prioritize cognitive or fine motor skills.

3. Common Conditions Treated with Physiotherapy:-

Physiotherapy is a healthcare treatment aimed at improving a person's movement, function, and overall well-being. It uses various physical methods such as exercises, manual therapy, massage, and the use of machines like ultrasound or heat therapy to treat a range of conditions. Here are some common conditions treated with physiotherapy:

1. Musculoskeletal Conditions:

-Back and Neck Pain: Physiotherapy can help reduce pain and improve mobility through exercises and manual therapy.

-Arthritis: Exercise programs and joint mobilizations can reduce stiffness and pain in arthritic joints.

-Sports Injuries: Rehab exercises, taping, and manual therapy can restore function and prevent re-injury.

2. Neurological Conditions:

-Stroke: Physiotherapy can aid in regaining movement and coordination through targeted exercises and mobility training.

- Multiple Sclerosis (MS): It helps manage fatigue, mobility, and strength in people with MS.

- Parkinson's Disease: Balance, coordination, and mobility exercises help improve function.

3. Respiratory Conditions:

-Chronic Obstructive Pulmonary Disease (COPD): Breathing exercises and chest physiotherapy can help improve lung function.

-Asthma: Techniques to strengthen respiratory muscles and manage breathing patterns are often used.

4. Post-Surgical Rehabilitation:-

- After surgeries like knee replacements or hip replacements, physiotherapy can help restore movement and strength in the affected areas.

5. Pediatric Conditions:

  - Conditions like cerebral palsy, delayed motor skills, and developmental issues can be treated with exercises and mobility training to improve coordination and strength.

6. Orthopedic Injuries:-

  - Fractures, sprains, and dislocations are managed with strengthening exercises, mobility restoration, and pain management.

Physiotherapists tailor treatment plans based on the individual's needs to help them recover and improve their quality of life.

A) Musculoskeletal conditions (e.g., arthritis, back pain):-

Musculoskeletal conditions are a broad category of diseases or disorders that affect the body's muscles, bones, joints, tendons, ligaments, and surrounding soft tissues. These conditions can result in pain, stiffness, swelling, and a decrease in mobility or function. They vary widely in severity, ranging from minor sprains to chronic conditions like osteoarthritis. Here is an in-depth explanation of some common musculoskeletal conditions:

1.Osteoarthritis (OA):-

  - **Description:** A degenerative joint disease characterized by the breakdown of cartilage, the tissue that cushions the ends of bones in joints.

  - **Causes:** Aging, joint injury, obesity, genetics, and overuse of joints.

  - **Symptoms:** Joint pain, stiffness, swelling, and decreased range of motion, particularly in weight-bearing joints like the knees, hips, and spine.

  - **Treatment:** Lifestyle changes (weight management, exercise), pain relief medications (NSAIDs, acetaminophen), physical therapy, and in severe cases, joint replacement surgery.

2.Rheumatoid Arthritis (RA) :-

Description: An autoimmune disease in which the body's immune system attacks the synovium (lining of the joints), causing inflammation and joint damage.

  - **Causes:** Exact causes are unknown, but genetic and environmental factors contribute.

  - **Symptoms:** Symmetrical joint pain, swelling, stiffness (especially in the morning), fatigue, and in advanced cases, joint deformity.

  - **Treatment:** Disease-modifying antirheumatic drugs (DMARDs), biologics, corticosteroids, pain relievers, and physical therapy.

3. Osteoporosis:-

  - **Description:** A condition in which bones become weak and brittle due to a loss of bone mass, increasing the risk of fractures.

-**Causes:** Aging, hormonal changes (especially in postmenopausal women), vitamin D and calcium deficiency, certain medications, and lifestyle factors (smoking, lack of exercise).

- **Symptoms:** Often no symptoms until a fracture occurs. Common fracture sites include the hip, spine, and wrist.

- **Treatment:** Calcium and vitamin D supplements, medications like bisphosphonates, hormone therapy, and weight-bearing exercises to strengthen bones.

4.Tendinitis:-

-**Description:** Inflammation or irritation of a tendon, the fibrous cord that attaches muscle to bone.

-**Causes:**Overuse or repetitive movements, injury, or aging.

- **Symptoms:** Pain and tenderness along a tendon, often near joints like the shoulder, elbow, knee, or ankle.

- **Treatment:** Rest, ice, physical therapy, anti-inflammatory medications, and in severe cases, corticosteroid injections or surgery.

5. Back Pain:-

- **Description:** Pain in the lower or upper back, often related to musculoskeletal issues such as muscle strain, disc problems, or spinal conditions.

- **Causes:** Poor posture, muscle strain, herniated discs, spinal stenosis, arthritis, or injury.

- **Symptoms:** Pain, stiffness, and limited range of motion, which may radiate to the legs (sciatica) in cases of nerve compression.

-**Treatment:** Pain relief medications, physical therapy, exercises, ergonomic adjustments, and in some cases, surgery (e.g., for herniated discs).

6. Fibromyalgia:

- **Description:** A chronic condition characterized by widespread musculoskeletal pain, along with fatigue, sleep disturbances, memory issues, and mood disorders.

- **Causes:**The exact cause is unclear but may involve abnormal pain processing in the brain, genetics, stress, and infections.

- **Symptoms:** Widespread pain, tenderness, fatigue, sleep problems, and cognitive difficulties (often called "fibro fog").

- **Treatment:** Pain relievers, antidepressants, anti-seizure medications, physical therapy, exercise, and stress management techniques.

7. Carpal Tunnel Syndrome:-

- **Description:** A condition caused by compression of the median nerve as it travels through the carpal tunnel in the wrist.

- **Causes:** Repetitive hand movements, wrist anatomy, pregnancy, and certain health conditions (e.g., diabetes, rheumatoid arthritis).

- **Symptoms:** Numbness, tingling, weakness, and pain in the hand and fingers, especially the thumb, index, and middle fingers.

- **Treatment:** Wrist splinting, avoiding repetitive movements, anti-inflammatory medications, corticosteroid injections, and surgery in severe cases.

8. Bursitis:-

- **Description:** Inflammation of the bursae, small fluid-filled sacs that cushion bones, tendons, and muscles near joints.

- **Causes:** Repetitive movements, prolonged pressure on a joint, injury, infection, or underlying conditions like arthritis.

- **Symptoms:** Pain, swelling, and tenderness in the affected area, often near joints like the shoulder, elbow, or hip.

- **Treatment:** Rest, ice, anti-inflammatory medications, physical therapy, and corticosteroid injections if necessary.

9.Scoliosis:-

- **Description:** An abnormal lateral curvature of the spine.

- **Causes**: The cause is often idiopathic (unknown), but can also be congenital, due to neuromuscular conditions, or related to degeneration in older adults.

- **Symptoms:** Uneven shoulders or hips, back pain, and in severe cases, breathing difficulties due to the compression of internal organs.

- **Treatment:** Observation, bracing (in growing children), and surgery for severe cases (spinal fusion).

10. Muscle Strain:-

- **Description:** Injury to a muscle or its tendons, often resulting from overstretching or overuse.

- **Causes:** Sudden heavy lifting, overstretching, fatigue, or lack of proper warm-up before exercise.

- **Symptoms:** Pain, swelling, muscle weakness, and limited movement.

- **Treatment:** Rest, ice, compression, elevation (R.I.C.E.), physical therapy, and gradual re-strengthening exercises.

Risk Factors for Musculoskeletal Conditions:-

- **Age:** Many musculoskeletal conditions, like osteoarthritis and osteoporosis, are more common with aging.

- **Physical Activity:** High-impact sports or repetitive movements increase the risk of conditions like tendinitis and bursitis.

- **Obesity:** Excess weight puts stress on joints, particularly in the lower body, contributing to conditions like osteoarthritis.

- **Genetics:** Some conditions, like rheumatoid arthritis or scoliosis, have a genetic predisposition.

- **Occupational Factors:** Jobs that involve heavy lifting, repetitive motions, or prolonged periods of sitting/standing can increase the risk of developing musculoskeletal disorders.

Prevention and Management:-

- **Regular Exercise:** Strength training, flexibility exercises, and aerobic activities help maintain muscle and joint health.

- **Proper Ergonomics:** Using proper posture and supportive equipment (e.g., ergonomic chairs) can reduce the strain on muscles and joints.

- **Healthy Diet:** Adequate intake of calcium and vitamin D is essential for bone health.

- **Weight Management:** Maintaining a healthy weight reduces stress on joints.

- **Early Diagnosis and Treatment:** Prompt medical attention can help manage symptoms and slow the progression of chronic musculoskeletal conditions.

Musculoskeletal conditions are a major cause of disability worldwide, but with proper management, many individuals can lead active, fulfilling lives.

B) Neurological conditions (e.g., stroke recovery, Parkinson's disease) :-

Neurological conditions refer to disorders that affect the brain, spinal cord, and nerves throughout the body. These conditions can result in a variety of symptoms, such as difficulties with movement, sensation, memory, cognition, and autonomic functions. Neurological disorders can be caused by a variety of factors, including genetic abnormalities, injury, infections, degenerative processes, and autoimmune responses. Here's a detailed exploration of common neurological conditions:

1. Stroke:-

- Description: A stroke occurs when the blood supply to part of the brain is interrupted or reduced, depriving brain tissue of oxygen and nutrients. This leads to the death of brain cells within minutes.

- **Causes:** Blockage of blood vessels (ischemic stroke), rupture of blood vessels (hemorrhagic stroke), or temporary reduction in blood flow (transient ischemic attack or TIA).

- **Symptoms:** Sudden weakness or numbness, especially on one side of the body, trouble speaking or understanding speech, vision problems, loss of coordination, and severe headache.

- **Treatment:** Emergency treatment includes clot-busting drugs for ischemic stroke, surgery to stop bleeding in hemorrhagic stroke, and rehabilitation to regain lost functions like speech or movement.

2. Parkinson's Disease:-

- **Description:** A progressive neurodegenerative disorder that affects movement, caused by the loss of dopamine-producing neurons in a specific area of the brain (substantia nigra).

- **Causes:** The exact cause is unknown, but a combination of genetic and environmental factors is believed to contribute.

- **Symptoms:** Tremors (shaking), bradykinesia (slowness of movement), muscle stiffness, impaired balance, and changes in speech and handwriting.

- **Treatment:** Medications to increase dopamine levels (e.g., levodopa), deep brain stimulation (DBS), and physical therapy to improve movement and coordination.

3.Multiple Sclerosis (MS) :-

- **Description:** A chronic autoimmune disorder where the immune system attacks the protective covering (myelin) of nerve fibers in the central nervous system, disrupting the communication between the brain and the rest of the body.

- **Causes:** The exact cause is unknown, but it's believed to involve genetic and environmental factors.

- **Symptoms:** Fatigue, difficulty walking, numbness or tingling, muscle weakness, vision problems, and difficulty with coordination and balance.

- **Treatment:** Disease-modifying therapies (DMTs) to slow progression, steroids to manage relapses, and therapies to manage specific symptoms (e.g., physical therapy, occupational therapy).

4. Alzheimer's Disease:-

- **Description:** A progressive neurodegenerative disease and the most common form of dementia, characterized by memory loss, confusion, and a decline in cognitive functions due to the death of brain cells.

- **Causes:**The accumulation of abnormal proteins (amyloid plaques and tau tangles) in the brain, along with genetic and environmental factors, are thought to contribute.

- **Symptoms:** Memory loss, difficulty with problem-solving, confusion with time or place, trouble speaking or writing, and changes in mood or behavior.

- **Treatment:** Medications such as cholinesterase inhibitors and memantine to manage symptoms, along with lifestyle changes and cognitive therapies to slow cognitive decline.

5. Epilepsy:-

- **Description:** A neurological disorder characterized by recurrent, unprovoked seizures, which are abnormal electrical discharges in the brain.

- **Causes:** Brain injury, genetic factors, infections, developmental disorders, or unknown causes (idiopathic epilepsy).

- **Symptoms:** Seizures can vary, ranging from brief lapses in attention or convulsions to loss of consciousness or muscle control.

- **Treatment:** Antiepileptic drugs (AEDs), surgery for patients who don't respond to medication, and in some cases, ketogenic diets or nerve stimulation therapies.

6. Migraine:-

- **Description:** A type of headache disorder that causes severe, throbbing pain, often accompanied by nausea, vomiting, and sensitivity to light and sound.

- **Causes:** While the exact cause is unclear, migraines are thought to involve genetic and environmental factors, including changes in brain activity and blood flow.

- **Symptoms:** Intense headache (often on one side), visual disturbances (aura), nausea, sensitivity to light, and fatigue. Migraine attacks can last hours to days.

- **Treatment:** Pain-relief medications (e.g., NSAIDs, triptans), preventative medications (e.g., beta-blockers, anticonvulsants), and lifestyle changes (e.g., stress management, diet changes).

7. Amyotrophic Lateral Sclerosis (ALS)

- **Description:** A progressive neurodegenerative disease that affects motor neurons in the brain and spinal cord, leading to muscle weakness, paralysis, and eventually death.

- **Causes:** While the cause is mostly unknown, genetic mutations are involved in a small percentage of cases.

- **Symptoms:** Muscle weakness, difficulty speaking and swallowing, and paralysis. ALS usually starts in the limbs and spreads to the rest of the body, eventually affecting breathing muscles.

- **Treatment:** Riluzole and edaravone are medications that may slow the progression of the disease, along with therapies to manage symptoms and maintain quality of life.

8. Peripheral Neuropathy:-

- **Description:** A condition that results from damage to the peripheral nerves, which can affect sensation, movement, and organ function.

- **Causes**: Diabetes (diabetic neuropathy), infections, injuries, vitamin deficiencies, toxins, and autoimmune diseases.

- **Symptoms:** Numbness, tingling, burning sensations, sharp pains, and muscle weakness, especially in the hands and feet.

- **Description:** Pain relief medications, management of the underlying cause (e.g., blood sugar control in diabetes), physical therapy, and in some cases, nerve stimulation or surgery.

9. Huntington's Disease:-

- **Description:** A genetic disorder that causes progressive degeneration of nerve cells in the brain, affecting movement, cognition, and psychiatric health.

- **Causes:** A mutation in the huntingtin gene, leading to the production of an abnormal protein that damages brain cells.

- **Symptoms:** Uncontrolled movements (chorea), cognitive decline, mood swings, and personality changes. Symptoms typically appear between the ages of 30 and 50.

- **Treatment:** While there's no cure, medications can help manage symptoms like chorea and psychiatric conditions, along with therapies for cognitive and physical functions.

10. Guillain-Barré Syndrome (GBS):-

- **Description:** A rare autoimmune disorder where the immune system attacks the peripheral nerves, leading to muscle weakness and, in severe cases, paralysis.

- **Causes:** Often triggered by an infection (e.g., respiratory or gastrointestinal infection), though the exact mechanism is unclear.

- **Symptoms:** Rapid-onset weakness, starting in the legs and progressing upward, tingling, and in severe cases, respiratory failure.

- **Treatment:** Immunoglobulin therapy (IVIg) or plasma exchange to reduce immune attack on the nerves, along with supportive care, physical therapy, and ventilatory support if needed.

11. Cerebral Palsy

- **Description:** A group of neurological disorders that appear in early childhood and affect movement, posture, and coordination due to damage to the developing brain.

- **Causes:** Brain injury or malformations during prenatal development, birth complications, or early childhood brain injuries.

- **Symptoms:** Motor impairments like spasticity, muscle weakness, coordination issues, and in some cases, intellectual disability, speech problems, and seizures.

- **Treatment:** Physical therapy, occupational therapy, speech therapy, medications for spasticity, and sometimes surgery to correct musculoskeletal deformities.

Risk Factors for Neurological Conditions:-

- **Genetics:** Many neurological conditions, like Huntington's disease or some types of epilepsy, have a genetic component.

- **Infections:** Some neurological disorders, like Guillain-Barré syndrome or meningitis, can be triggered by infections.

- **Age:** The risk for neurodegenerative diseases, such as Alzheimer's and Parkinson's, increases with age.

- **Head Trauma:** Traumatic brain injuries can lead to conditions like epilepsy or long-term cognitive issues.

- **Environmental Factors:** Exposure to toxins, stress, poor nutrition, or lifestyle factors like smoking can contribute to the development of neurological conditions.

Prevention and Management:-

- **Healthy Lifestyle:** Regular exercise, a balanced diet, stress management, and avoidance of smoking and excessive alcohol consumption can reduce the risk of many neurological conditions.

- **Early Intervention:** Prompt diagnosis and treatment of conditions like stroke, epilepsy, and MS can slow progression and improve outcomes.

- **Ongoing Care:** Many neurological conditions require long-term management, including medications, therapies, and lifestyle adaptations to maintain quality of life.

Neurological conditions can have a profound impact on a person's quality of life, but with proper management, many patients can continue to lead fulfilling lives. Early detection, medical intervention, and support from healthcare professionals are key to managing symptoms and maintaining function.

C) Cardiopulmonary issues (e.g., COPD, post-surgery recovery) :-

Cardiopulmonary issues refer to problems affecting both the heart (cardio) and the lungs (pulmonary). These two organs work closely together to circulate oxygen-rich blood throughout the body. Any dysfunction in either the heart or lungs can lead to significant health problems, as they are essential for delivering oxygen and removing carbon dioxide from the blood.

Common Cardiopulmonary Issues:-

1.Heart Failure: This condition occurs when the heart cannot pump blood effectively, leading to inadequate circulation of oxygen and nutrients. Symptoms include shortness of breath, fatigue, and fluid buildup (edema) in the lungs, which makes breathing difficult.

2.Chronic Obstructive Pulmonary Disease (COPD): A lung condition that obstructs airflow, making it hard to breathe. Chronic bronchitis and emphysema are part of COPD. Over time, COPD can strain the heart, leading to cardiopulmonary complications.

3.Pulmonary Hypertension: High blood pressure in the lungs' arteries causes the right side of the heart to work harder to pump blood through the lungs. Over time, this can lead to heart failure. Symptoms include chest pain, shortness of breath, and fatigue.

4.Pulmonary Embolism : A blood clot that travels to the lungs, blocking a pulmonary artery. This condition can be life-threatening as it prevents the lungs from properly oxygenating the blood. Symptoms include sudden chest pain, rapid heartbeat, and shortness of breath.

5.Asthma : A chronic condition that causes the airways to narrow and become inflamed, leading to difficulty breathing. Severe asthma attacks can stress the heart, leading to cardiopulmonary complications.

6.Acute Respiratory Distress Syndrome (ARDS):- A life-threatening condition that leads to fluid buildup in the alveoli (air sacs) of the lungs, severely reducing the lungs' ability to oxygenate the blood. This can result from trauma, pneumonia, or sepsis, and often requires mechanical ventilation.
7. **Cor Pulmonale:** A condition where chronic lung disease (like COPD) leads to the enlargement and failure of the right side of the heart. It's a specific form of heart failure caused by lung disease.

Causes of Cardiopulmonary Issues:-

- Smoking : Major risk factor for both heart and lung diseases, including COPD, heart disease, and pulmonary hypertension.

- Obesity : Increases the risk of developing heart disease and breathing issues due to pressure on the lungs and heart.

- High Blood Pressure (Hypertension): Forces the heart to work harder, leading to heart disease and pulmonary hypertension.

- Infections : Conditions like pneumonia can lead to ARDS or exacerbate existing heart or lung problems.

- Air Pollution : Exposure to pollutants can damage the lungs and lead to chronic respiratory diseases, which affect heart function.

Symptoms of Cardiopulmonary Issues :-

- **Shortness of Breath** : A common symptom caused by either heart failure or lung disease.

- **Chest Pain** : Indicates heart issues like heart attacks, pulmonary embolism, or pulmonary hypertension.

- **Fatigue** : Lack of oxygen due to poor heart or lung function leads to tiredness.

- **Swelling in Legs or Abdomen** : A sign of heart failure, as the heart struggles to pump blood efficiently.

- **Rapid or Irregular Heartbeat** : May occur when the heart is strained due to pulmonary hypertension or other conditions.

Diagnosis:-

1.**Electrocardiogram (ECG):** Measures the electrical activity of the heart to detect heart disease.

2. **Chest X-Ray** : Helps identify lung conditions like COPD, pneumonia, or ARDS.

3. **Echocardiogram:** An ultrasound of the heart to assess its function and look for abnormalities.

4. **Pulmonary Function Tests (PFTs):** Measure lung capacity and airflow to diagnose lung diseases.

5. **Blood Gas Analysis:** Measures oxygen and carbon dioxide levels in the blood to assess lung function.

6. **CT Scan:** Provides detailed images of the heart and lungs to detect conditions like pulmonary embolism or tumors.

Treatment Approaches:-

1. Medications:

  - **Diuretics** to reduce fluid buildup in heart failure.

  - **Bronchodilators** to open airways in asthma or COPD.

  - **Anticoagulants** to prevent blood clots in pulmonary embolism.

2. Lifestyle Changes:

  - Quitting smoking, maintaining a healthy weight, and regular exercise are critical in managing cardiopulmonary conditions.

3. Oxygen Therapy: For individuals with advanced lung disease, oxygen therapy may be necessary to improve blood oxygen levels.

4. Surgical Interventions :

  - **Bypass Surgery or Angioplasty** to restore blood flow in blocked heart arteries.

  - **Lung Transplant** for severe, end-stage lung diseases like COPD or ARDS.

  - **Pulmonary Thromboendarterectomy** to remove blood clots from pulmonary arteries in severe pulmonary hypertension.

Prevention:-

- **Healthy Diet:** A heart-healthy diet rich in fruits, vegetables, and lean proteins helps prevent cardiovascular disease.

- **Regular Exercise:** Improves both heart and lung function.

- **Vaccinations :** Staying up-to-date on vaccines like the flu shot and pneumonia vaccine reduces the risk of respiratory infections.

- **Avoiding Smoking and Pollutants:** Reduces the risk of developing COPD, lung cancer, and other lung diseases.

Managing cardiopulmonary issues requires a multidisciplinary approach, involving lifestyle changes, medication, and sometimes advanced medical or surgical interventions. Early diagnosis and treatment are key to improving outcomes.

D) Pediatric physiotherapy (e.g., cerebral palsy) :-

Pediatric physiotherapy, also known as pediatric physical therapy, is a specialized branch of physiotherapy focused on assessing, treating, and managing children from infancy through adolescence who experience physical difficulties related to movement, coordination, balance, strength, and developmental delays. The goal of pediatric physiotherapy is to help children achieve their optimal physical development and improve their quality of life by addressing any physical challenges they may face.

Key Areas of Pediatric Physiotherapy:-

1. **Developmental Delays:**

   - Some children experience delays in reaching key milestones, such as rolling over, sitting, standing, crawling, and walking. Pediatric physiotherapists work with these children to promote the development of gross motor skills.

   2. **Neurological Conditions:**

   - Conditions like **cerebral palsy, spina bifida, muscular dystrophy**, and **Down syndrome** affect the nervous system, leading to movement and coordination challenges. Pediatric physiotherapists use exercises, stretching, and specialized equipment to improve the child's mobility, balance, and strength.

3. **Musculoskeletal Conditions:**

   - Children may develop musculoskeletal issues such as **scoliosis, torticollis (neck muscle tightness)**, or **joint hypermobility**. Pediatric physiotherapists address these issues by strengthening muscles, correcting postural problems, and improving flexibility.

4.Orthopedic Rehabilitation:

   - Pediatric physiotherapy can be essential following fractures, sports injuries, or surgeries. Therapists help children regain strength, mobility, and flexibility in the affected areas, using age-appropriate methods.

   5. **Respiratory Conditions:**

   - Pediatric physiotherapists work with children who have respiratory conditions such as **cystic fibrosis, asthma, and bronchopulmonary dysplasia**. They use techniques such as chest physiotherapy to clear the airways and improve lung function.

6. Congenital and Genetic Conditions:

   - Children born with conditions like **clubfoot, Erb's palsy (nerve injury during birth),** or **osteogenesis imperfecta** (brittle bone disease) may require long-term physiotherapy to manage symptoms and improve function.

7. Premature Birth:

   - Babies born prematurely often require physiotherapy to assist with developmental milestones, coordination, muscle tone, and respiratory function due to the early challenges they face.

8. Sensory Processing Disorders:

   - Children with sensory integration issues, often found in conditions like **autism spectrum disorder**, may benefit from physiotherapy to improve balance, coordination, and body awareness through movement-based activities.

   ****Key Techniques and Approaches in Pediatric Physiotherapy: ****

1. Play-Based Therapy

   - Play is central to pediatric physiotherapy because children learn and engage better through play. Therapeutic exercises are often disguised as games or fun activities to keep children motivated and involved. For example, balance exercises might involve obstacle courses, and strengthening activities may include lifting toys.

2. Motor Skill Development:

   - Therapists focus on improving gross motor skills (e.g., crawling, walking, running) and fine motor skills (e.g., hand-eye coordination) using tailored exercises that target specific muscle groups and movements.

3. Stretching and Strengthening Exercises:

   - For children with tight muscles or weakness, stretching and strengthening exercises help improve flexibility, posture, and overall mobility. These exercises can be incorporated into everyday routines and may include activities such as squats, lunges, or yoga-based movements.

4. Postural Training:

   - Postural alignment is essential for proper movement. Therapists help children develop better posture, which can be especially beneficial for those with conditions like scoliosis or cerebral palsy.

5. Balance and Coordination Training:

   - To improve balance and coordination, therapists may use exercises like standing on one foot, walking on balance beams, or using wobble boards and other equipment. This is particularly important for children with developmental delays or neurological conditions.

6. Taping and Orthotics:

   - Some children benefit from supportive devices such as **orthotic braces** or **kinesiology taping**. These tools help support weak muscles, correct alignment, and improve movement patterns.

7. Hydrotherapy:

   - Water-based therapy, or hydrotherapy, is an effective method for treating children, especially those with limited mobility or muscle weakness. The buoyancy of water supports the body, making it easier for children to move and exercise without placing too much strain on their joints.

8. Respiratory Physiotherapy Techniques:

   - Children with respiratory conditions may require specific techniques such as chest percussions, vibrations, postural drainage, and breathing exercises to help clear mucus from the lungs and improve their breathing patterns.

Conditions Treated by Pediatric Physiotherapists:

1.**Cerebral Palsy (CP):** A neurological disorder affecting muscle tone, movement, and motor skills. Pediatric physiotherapists work on improving muscle strength, posture, balance, and functional movement in children with CP.

2.**Developmental Coordination Disorder (DCD):** Also known as dyspraxia, DCD affects a child's ability to coordinate movements. Physiotherapy focuses on improving motor skills and coordination to make everyday activities easier.

3.**Torticollis:** A condition where the neck muscles are tight on one side, leading to a head tilt. Physiotherapy helps to stretch the tight muscles and improve head movement.

7. Spina Bifida : A congenital condition where the spinal cord does not develop properly. Physiotherapists help children with spina bifida strengthen their muscles, improve mobility, and, when needed, adapt to assistive devices.

Scoliosis: An abnormal curvature of the spine that often develops in adolescence. Pediatric physiotherapy aims to improve posture, prevent further progression, and strengthen the back muscles.

Clubfoot: A congenital condition where one or both feet are twisted inward. Early physiotherapy, often combined with casting or surgery, helps correct the foot's position and improves function.

Down Syndrome: Children with Down syndrome often have low muscle tone and joint hypermobility. Physiotherapy focuses on improving muscle strength, balance, and coordination to help these children achieve motor milestones.

Autism Spectrum Disorder (ASD): Many children with ASD have sensory processing issues, motor delays, and poor balance. Pediatric physiotherapists help improve these areas through sensory-motor activities and structured play.

Role of Parents and Caregivers:-

Parental involvement is crucial in pediatric physiotherapy. Therapists often educate parents and caregivers on how to support their child's physical development at home by incorporating therapeutic exercises into daily routines. Consistency between therapy sessions and at-home activities is key to successful outcomes.

Benefits of Pediatric Physiotherapy:-

1. Improved Mobility and Independence: Children gain strength, coordination, and movement skills, allowing them to participate more fully in everyday activities and achieve greater independence.

2. Enhanced Quality of Life: Physiotherapy helps children overcome physical challenges, reducing pain and discomfort, improving self-confidence, and enhancing their ability to play and interact with others.

3.Prevention of Secondary Complications: Early intervention helps prevent complications such as muscle stiffness, joint deformities, and loss of function that could arise from untreated physical conditions.

4.Faster Recovery: After injury or surgery, pediatric physiotherapy promotes faster and more effective recovery by targeting areas that need rehabilitation and strengthening.

5.Social and Emotional Development: Participating in fun, interactive activities during physiotherapy also supports children's social and emotional development, building positive experiences and relationships.

Pediatric physiotherapy plays an essential role in supporting children with various physical and developmental challenges, enabling them to reach their fullest potential in movement and overall well-being.

E)Geriatric physiotherapy for elderly individuals :-

Geriatric physiotherapy focuses on addressing the physical health concerns and mobility issues of elderly individuals. As people age, they experience changes in muscle strength, joint mobility, balance, and coordination, which can lead to a decline in functional independence. Geriatric physiotherapy aims to improve or maintain physical function, reduce pain, and enhance the overall quality of life in older adults.

1.Common Age-Related Conditions Addressed:

Elderly individuals often face multiple age-related issues that physiotherapy can help manage:

- **Osteoarthritis:** Joint stiffness and pain, especially in weight-bearing joints like the knees and hips.

- **Osteoporosis:** Loss of bone density, leading to an increased risk of fractures, especially in the spine, hips, and wrists.

- **Balance and Fall Prevention:** Elderly people are prone to falls due to weakened muscles, poor vision, or neurological issues.

- **Postural Instability:** Poor posture from spinal degeneration or muscle weakness can lead to functional limitations.

- **Neurological Disorders:** Conditions like Parkinson's disease, stroke, and dementia, which affect mobility and coordination.

- **Post-Surgical Recovery:** Rehabilitation after surgeries like joint replacements, fractures, or cardiovascular surgeries.

2. Goals of Geriatric Physiotherapy:

- **Enhance Mobility and Independence:** Physiotherapists work on improving the mobility of the elderly, focusing on walking, climbing stairs, and other daily activities.

- **Strengthen Muscles:** Weak muscles can affect balance and cause joint pain, so physiotherapy helps in improving muscle strength through exercises.

- **Improve Balance and Coordination:** Balance training is critical to reducing the risk of falls and ensuring safety.

- **Reduce Pain:** Techniques like manual therapy, heat therapy, or electrical stimulation help reduce chronic pain conditions.

- **Improve Cardiovascular Fitness:** Exercise routines are often designed to improve cardiovascular health, especially for those recovering from surgeries or living with conditions like heart disease.

- **Enhance Flexibility:** Stretching exercises are introduced to improve joint mobility and flexibility, especially in the hips, spine, and shoulders.

3.Assessment and Individualized Treatment

A physiotherapist begins by conducting a thorough assessment of the individual's current physical capabilities, medical history, and specific conditions. Based on this, an individualized treatment plan is created, which might include:

- **Functional Exercises:** Exercises to improve balance, coordination, and walking.

- **Strength Training:** Targeted exercises for major muscle groups, focusing on the legs, arms, and core.

- **Range of Motion Exercises:** Movements to improve flexibility and reduce joint stiffness.

- **Manual Therapy:** Techniques like massage, joint mobilization, and soft tissue manipulation to reduce pain and improve mobility.

- **Assistive Devices:** Education and training on using assistive devices like walkers, canes, or orthotics to enhance safety and mobility.

4.Techniques Used in Geriatric Physiotherapy:

- **Therapeutic Exercises:** Tailored to the individual's ability, these exercises aim to restore strength, flexibility, and endurance.

- **Hydrotherapy:** Water-based exercises that are gentle on the joints, helping with conditions like arthritis.

- **Electrotherapy:** The use of electrical stimulation (e.g., TENS) to relieve pain and improve muscle function.

- **Postural Training:** Exercises that focus on improving posture to prevent falls, reduce back pain, and promote alignment.

- **Gait Training:** Focused exercises and practices to improve walking patterns and reduce fall risks.

5.Benefits of Geriatric Physiotherapy:

- **Increased Independence:** Physiotherapy can help older adults perform daily activities with less assistance, allowing them to stay active and independent.

- **Pain Relief:** For those suffering from conditions like arthritis, physiotherapy can reduce chronic pain and discomfort.

- **Prevention of Falls:** By improving strength, balance, and coordination, physiotherapy significantly reduces the risk of falls.

- **Improved Mental Health:** Physical improvements often lead to increased self-esteem and a better overall sense of well-being.

- **Enhanced Quality of Life:** The ability to move freely without pain or fear of injury contributes to an enhanced quality of life for elderly individuals.

6.Home Exercises and Education:

Physiotherapists often teach patients and caregivers home exercises that can be continued outside of therapy sessions. Education is also provided to ensure elderly individuals know how to manage their conditions and reduce injury risks.

7. Multidisciplinary Approach:

Geriatric physiotherapy is often part of a broader healthcare approach, involving physicians, occupational therapists, and caregivers. A multidisciplinary approach ensures comprehensive care, addressing not only physical but also psychological and emotional aspects of aging.

8. Cognitive and Emotional Support:

Some elderly patients may suffer from conditions like dementia or depression, which can affect their ability to follow physiotherapy. A skilled physiotherapist tailors the approach to suit the cognitive and emotional state of the patient, ensuring that treatment remains compassionate and patient-centered.

In conclusion, geriatric physiotherapy plays a vital role in helping elderly individuals maintain their independence, manage chronic pain, and improve their physical and emotional well-being.

4. Benefits of Physiotherapy for General Population:-

Physiotherapy offers numerous benefits to the general population, improving overall health, mobility and quality of life.

A) Improved mobility and flexibility:

Improving mobility and flexibility in physiotherapy is crucial for patients recovering from injury, surgery, or managing chronic conditions. Mobility refers to the ability to move freely and easily, while flexibility is the range of motion in the joints and muscles. Here are some key strategies used in physiotherapy to enhance both:

1.Stretching Exercises:-

  - **Static Stretching:** Holding a muscle in a stretched position for 15-60 seconds helps improve flexibility over time.

  - **Dynamic Stretching:**

Controlled, active movements that take muscles through their full range of motion, often used as a warm-up to enhance mobility.

  - **PNF Stretching (Proprioceptive Neuromuscular Facilitation):** Involves alternating between stretching and contracting muscles to increase range of motion.

2.Strengthening Exercises:-

  - Strengthening muscles around the joints can improve stability and support better movement. Stronger muscles help reduce stiffness and enhance joint flexibility.

  - Exercises like squats, lunges, and resistance band work can build strength in key muscle groups.

3. Manual Therapy:-

  - **Joint Mobilization:** A hands-on technique where the therapist gently moves the joint to increase its range of motion.

  - **Soft Tissue Mobilization:** Massaging or manipulating the soft tissues (muscles, tendons, and ligaments) to reduce tightness and improve flexibility.

4.Range of Motion (ROM) Exercises:-

   - Passive, active, or assisted ROM exercises are used to help joints move through their full range, often following surgery or injury to prevent stiffness.

   - These exercises are tailored to the patient's condition, ensuring gradual improvement.

  5. Functional Training:-

   - Incorporating movements that mimic everyday activities, like walking, reaching, or bending, to improve overall mobility.

   - Focuses on improving coordination, balance, and muscle activation.

  6. Neuromuscular Re-education:-

Helps retrain the nervous system and muscles to work together effectively after injury or surgery, improving movement patterns and overall mobility.

  7. Hydrotherapy:-

Water exercises provide a low-impact environment where patients can move more freely, reducing strain on joints and muscles while still working on mobility and flexibility.

  8. Foam Rolling and Myofascial Release:-

   - Foam rolling helps release tension in the fascia (connective tissue surrounding muscles), increasing flexibility and reducing muscle tightness.

   - Myofascial release is a manual technique that involves applying gentle pressure to fascia to restore movement.

  9. Postural Training:-

   - Improving posture can relieve unnecessary tension on muscles and joints, which can lead to better mobility and flexibility.

   - Postural corrections help align the body properly, reducing stiffness and enhancing movement efficiency.

  10. Yoga and Pilates:-

   - Both methods combine stretching, strength training, and controlled breathing to promote flexibility, balance, and mobility.

   - These techniques are often integrated into physiotherapy programs to enhance joint range and muscle elongation.

By combining these approaches, physiotherapists create personalized plans to address a patient's specific mobility and flexibility needs, ensuring they can regain or maintain an active, pain-free lifestyle.

B) Pain management without medication:-

Pain management without medication in physiotherapy can be effectively achieved through a combination of techniques that focus on physical, mental, and behavioral approaches. Here are some common non-pharmacological methods used:

1. Exercise Therapy:-

  - **Strengthening & Stretching** : Targeted exercises can strengthen weak muscles, improve posture, and reduce pain. Stretching improves flexibility and reduces muscle tension.

  - **Aerobic Exercises** : Low-impact activities like swimming, walking, and cycling improve blood flow and reduce stiffness.

2. Manual Therapy:-

  - **Massage:** Helps relax tight muscles, improve circulation, and reduce inflammation.

  - **Joint Mobilization/Manipulation** : Aimed at restoring movement in joints, this technique can relieve pain and stiffness.

3.Heat and Cold Therapy:-

 Heat Therapy : Increases blood flow, relaxes muscles, and improves tissue elasticity. Used for chronic conditions.

 Cold Therapy : Reduces inflammation, swelling, and numbs acute pain. Ideal for injuries and swelling.

4. Electrical Stimulation (TENS):-

Transcutaneous Electrical Nerve Stimulation (TENS) :Uses low-voltage electrical currents to interfere with pain signals sent to the brain, offering temporary relief.

5. Ultrasound Therapy:-

Uses sound waves to penetrate tissues, reducing inflammation, improving blood flow, and accelerating healing in soft tissues.

6.Dry Needling:-

A technique where fine needles are inserted into trigger points or areas of muscle tightness to alleviate pain and improve movement.

7.Hydrotherapy:-

Water-based exercises help reduce joint strain, improve muscle tone, and alleviate pain due to the buoyancy of water.

8.Posture Correction:-

Focusing on ergonomic modifications and exercises that correct poor posture can prevent pain related to bad alignment, particularly in the spine and shoulders.

9.Cognitive Behavioral Therapy (CBT):-

Though not a physical technique, CBT is used in physiotherapy to help patients change their pain perception and improve coping mechanisms.

10. Mind-Body Techniques:-

Breathing exercises, relaxation techniques, and guided imagery are used to manage stress and reduce pain perception.

11.Kinesio Taping:-

Elastic therapeutic tape is applied to support muscles and joints, reducing pain and inflammation, and enhancing movement.

These techniques are often customized depending on the individual's condition, tolerance, and overall rehabilitation goals. Physiotherapists typically incorporate multiple modalities for optimal pain relief and functional improvement.

C) Injury prevention:-

Injury prevention in physiotherapy focuses on strengthening the body, improving flexibility, and promoting proper movement patterns. Here are some key principles:

- **Warm-up** : Always start with a proper warm-up, like light aerobic exercises, to increase blood flow to muscles and reduce injury risk.

- **Strengthening muscles** : Focus on building strength, especially in core and stabilizing muscles, to support joints and maintain proper alignment during activity.

- **Flexibility** : Regular stretching improves flexibility, reducing muscle tightness and improving range of motion.

- **Correct posture and technique** : Using proper posture and movement techniques during exercises and daily activities helps prevent strain and injury.
- **Balance and coordination:** Training for balance and coordination reduces the risk of falls and joint injuries, especially in dynamic sports.
- **Adequate rest:** Rest is essential for recovery, allowing muscles and tissues to repair and prevent overuse injuries.

- **Gradual progression** : Avoid sudden increases in intensity or duration of exercise to prevent overloading muscles and joints.

- **Use proper footwear and equipment:** Wearing supportive shoes and using appropriate equipment can reduce the risk of injury.

These guidelines, combined with regular check-ins with a physiotherapist, can significantly lower the risk of injuries.

D) Better posture and body mechanics :-

Improving posture and body mechanics can significantly enhance your physical well-being, reducing the risk of injury and discomfort. Here are some tips to help:

1. Standing Posture

- **Align your ears, shoulders, hips, knees, and ankles:** Imagine a straight line running from your ears through your shoulders and hips down to your ankles.

- **Distribute your weight evenly:** Stand with your feet shoulder-width apart, and avoid shifting weight to one leg for too long.

- **Engage your core:** A strong core helps stabilize your body and maintain proper posture.

- **Avoid locking your knees:** Keep a slight bend to reduce pressure on the joints.

2. Sitting Posture

- **Sit with your back straight:** Keep your back supported, and avoid slumping.

- Adjust your chair so that your feet are flat on the floor or on a footrest.

- **Keep your shoulders relaxed:** Avoid rounding your shoulders forward. Keep them back and relaxed.

- **Position your screen at eye level:** If working at a computer, ensure that the monitor is at or slightly below eye level to prevent neck strain.

3. Lifting Mechanics

- **Bend at the knees, not the waist:** Use your legs, not your back, to lift heavy objects.

- **Keep objects close to your body:** This helps reduce the strain on your back and prevent injury.

- **Lift with your legs and tighten your core:** Squat to pick up objects and engage your abdominal muscles for extra support.

4. Walking Posture:-

- **Stand tall with your chin parallel to the floor:** Avoid looking down at your feet.

- **Relax your shoulders and swing your arms naturally:** This helps maintain Use a supportive mattress: Ensure that your spine maintains its natural alignment.

- **Sleep on your back or side:** Avoid sleeping on your stomach as it can cause neck and back strain.

- **Use a pillow to support your neck and spine:** A pillow that keeps your head in line with your body can prevent neck pain.

Consistent practice of these habits can lead to better overall posture and long-term health benefits.

E) Mental health benefits (reduced stress, anxiety):-

The benefits of good mental health are extensive and can enhance both your emotional well-being and overall quality of life. Here are some key benefits:

1. Improved Emotional Resilience:

Good mental health helps you cope with stress, anxiety, and life's challenges more effectively. You're better equipped to handle adversity and bounce back from setbacks.

2. Enhanced Relationships: Positive mental health allows for better communication, empathy, and emotional intimacy, which strengthens personal and professional relationships.

3. Increased Productivity: When mentally healthy, your focus, decision-making, and problem-solving skills improve, boosting your productivity at work or in school.

4. Better Physical Health: Mental health is closely tied to physical health. Lower stress levels can reduce the risk of chronic conditions like heart disease, improve immune function, and promote better sleep.

5. Increased Self-Esteem: Good mental health often leads to higher self-esteem and confidence, which of stairs a positive self-image and encourages you to take on new challenges.

6. Improved Mood and Happiness: mental health helps in developing and utilizing healthier ways to deal with life's stresses and negative emotions, like practicing mindfulness, exercise, or seeking social support.

8. Reduced Risk of Mental Health Disorders: Maintaining mental well-being through regular self-care and stress management techniques can lower the risk of developing mental health disorders like depression or anxiety.

Investing in mental health has long-lasting, life-enriching rewards that can influence every aspect of your life.

5. Physiotherapy for Common Injuries:-

A) Sports injuries (sprains, ligament tears):-

Sports injuries are common among athletes and active individuals. They occur when excessive force is placed on muscles, bones, tendons, or joints. Here are key details about common sports injuries:

1. Sprains:-

• **Definition:** Damage to ligaments (tissue connecting bones).

• **Common Sites:** Ankles, knees, wrists.

• **Symptoms:** Pain, swelling, bruising, inability to move or bear weight.

• **Treatment:** Rest, Ice, Compression, Elevation (RICE), physical therapy, sometimes surgery for severe cases.

2. Strains:-

• **Definition:** Stretching or tearing of muscles or tendons.

• **Common Sites:** Hamstrings, lower back, groin.

• **Symptoms:** Pain, muscle spasms, swelling, limited motion.

Treatment: RICE, stretching, strengthening exercises, and rest.

3. Fractures (Broken Bones)

• **Definition:** Break or crack in a bone. Common Sites: Arms, legs, collarbone, wrist.

• **Symptoms:** Severe pain, swelling, deformity, inability to move the limb.

- **Treatment:** Immobilization (casts or splints), surgery for severe cases, physical therapy after healing.

4. Dislocations:-

- **Definition:** A joint is forced out of its normal position.
- **Common Sites:** Shoulders, knees,**fingers.**
- **Symptoms:** Intense pain, swelling, visible deformity, immobility.
- **Treatment:** Relocation by a medical professional, immobilization, and rehabilitation.

5. Tendinitis

- **Definition:** Inflammation of a tendon, usually due to overuse.
- **Common Sites:** Shoulders, elbows, knees, Achilles tendon.
- **Symptoms:** Pain, swelling, tenderness,reduced flexibility.
- **Treatment:** Rest, anti-inflammatory medications, physical therapy.

6. Concussions

- **Definition: Brain injury caused by a blow to the head or violent shaking.**
- **Common in: Contact sports like football, hockey, boxing.**
- **Symptoms: Headaches, confusion, dizziness, nausea, memory loss.**
- **Treatment: Rest, gradual return to activity, medical supervision to prevent complications.**

7. Shin Splints

- **Definition:** Pain along the shinbone (tibia) due to overuse.
- **Common in:** Runners, dancers.
- **Symptoms:** Sharp or throbbing pain,tenderness along the shin.
- **Treatment:**

8. Knee Injuries

- **Types: Includes ligament tears (ACL, MCL), meniscus tears, and patellar tendinitis.**
- **Symptoms:** Pain, instability, swelling, difficulty moving the knee.
- **Treatment:** Physical therapy, bracing,surgery (for severe ligament tears).

9. Rotator Cuff Injuries

- **Definition:** Damage to the muscles and tendons that stabilize the shoulder.
- **Common in:** Throwing sports, swimming, tennis.
- **Symptoms:** Pain, weakness, limited range of motion in the shoulder.
- **Treatmentte:** Rest, strengthening exercises, surgery for tears.

10. Achilles Tendon Injuries

• **Definition: Damage to the Achilles tendon, often caused by sudden movement or overuse.**

• **Symptoms:** Sharp pain at the back of the ankle, swelling, difficulty walking.

• **Treatment:** Rest, ice, physical therapy, and in severe cases, surgery. between training sessions to prevent overuse injuries.

• **Protective Gear:** Use appropriate gear, such as helmets, pads, and braces.

Consulting a healthcare professional for proper diagnosis and treatment is critical if you suspect a sports injury.

B) Work-related injuries (repetitive strain injury):-

Work-related injuries occur during the course of employment and can result. from accidents, repetitive stress, or hazardous work environments. Here are some common types and details of work-related injuries:

1. Slips, Trips, and Falls

• **Definition:** Injuries from losing balance due to wet floors, uneven surfaces, or obstacles.

• **Common Sites:** Construction sites, warehouses, offices. Injuries: Fractures, sprains, head injuries, back injuries.

• **Prevention:** Ensure clean, dry floors: proper lighting; non-slip footwear, and warning signs for hazards.

2. Repetitive Strain Injuries (RSI)

• **Definition:** Injuries from performing the same motion repeatedly, leading to muscle or joint damage.

• **Common Examples:** Carpal tunnel syndrome, tendonitis, bursitis. Affected Areas: Wrists, hands, shoulders, back.

• **Prevention:** Regular breaks, ergonomic workstations, stretching, proper posture.

3. Falls from Heights

• **Definition:** Falls from ladders, scaffolding, or rooftops. Common in: Construction, roofing, window cleaning.

• **Injuries:** Fractures, spinal injuries, traumatic brain injuries.

• **Prevention:** Use of harnesses, guardrails, and secure ladders; safety training.

4. Back Injuries

• **Definition:** Strains or herniated discs due to heavy lifting, poor posture, or repetitive bending.

• **Common in:** Warehousing, nursing, construction.

- **Injuries:** Lower back pain, slipped discs, sciatica.

- **Prevention:** Proper lifting techniques, mechanical aids, regular stretching.

5. Being Struck by Objects

- **Definition:** Injuries caused by falling tools, machinery, or materials.

- **Common in:** Warehouses, construction, manufacturing.

- **Injuries:** Head injuries, fractures, bruises.

- **Prevention:** Use of hard hats, proper storage of materials, safety barriers.

6. Machine-Related Injuries

- **Definition:** Injuries from improper use of machinery or malfunctioning equipment.

- **Common in:** Factories, workshops, agriculture.

- **Injuries:** Cuts, amputations, crush injuries, burns.

- **Prevention:** Machine guards, regular maintenance, proper training.

7. Vehicle-Related Accidents

- **Definition:** Accidents involving company vehicles, forklifts, or heavy machinery.

- **Common in:** Delivery jobs, construction, warehousing.

Injuries: Whiplash, fractures, head injuries.

- **Prevention:** Seatbelts, defensive driving training, regular vehicle maintenance.

8. Electrocution

- **Definition:** Injuries caused by contact with live electrical wires or equipment. Common in: Construction, electrical work, maintenance.

- **Injuries:** Burns, cardiac arrest, nerve damage.

- **Prevention:** Lockout/tagout procedures, protective gear, proper insulation.

9. Exposure to Harmful Substances

- **Definition:** Illness or injury caused by contact with chemicals, asbestos, fumes, or other hazardous materials

- **Common in:** Laboratories, manufacturing, agriculture.

- **Injuries:** Respiratory issues, skin irritation, chemical burns, cancer. Prevention: Proper ventilation, use of personal protective equipment (PPE), and safety training.

10. Hearing Loss

Definition: Damage to hearing due to prolonged exposure to loud noises in the workplace.

Common in: Construction, manufacturing, airports.

Symptoms: Ringing in the ears (tinnitus), partial or complete hearingloss. Prevention: Use of ear protection, regular noise monitoring, limiting exposure.

11. Burns

- **Definition:** Injuries caused by exposure to heat, chemicals, or electricity.
- **Common in:** Kitchen work, manufacturing, construction.
- **Injuries:** Thermal burns, chemical burns, electrical burns.
- **Prevention:** Use of protective gear, proper handling of hazardous substances, fire safety protocols.

12. Occupational Illnesses

- **Definition:** Long-term health issues caused by exposure to harmful substances or environments over time.
- **Examples:** Asbestosis, mesothelioma,silicosis, lead poisoning.
- **Common in:** Mining, construction, manufacturing, healthcare.
- **Prevention:** Use of PPE, regular health screenings, limiting exposure, following safety protocols.

Prevention and Safety Measures:-

- **Training:** Regular safety training for employees to recognize and avoid hazards.
- **Ergonomics:** Designing workstations to minimize strain on the body.
- **Personal Protective Equipment (PPE):** Helmets, gloves, safety glasses, and other gear to reduce injury risks.
- **Regular Breaks:** Encouraging rest to prevent fatigue and overuse injuries.
- **Workplace Safety Audits:** Regular inspections to identify and correct potential hazards.

Employers are typically required by law to maintain safe working conditions and

provide compensation for injuries that occur on the job.

C) Post-operative rehabilitation:-

Post-operative rehabilitation is a critical phase in the recovery process following surgery. It aims to restore function, minimize pain, and reduce the risk of complications. Rehabilitation plans vary based on the type of surgery, the patient's condition, and overall health.

1. Goals of Post-Operative Rehabilitation:-

- **Restore Mobility and Function:** Focuses on improving strength, flexibility, and range of motion in the operated area.
- **Pain Management:** Utilizing medications, physical therapy, and other modalities to control pain.
- **Prevent Complications:** Such as infections, blood clots, or muscle atrophy.
- **Psychological Support:** Helping patients cope with stress, anxiety, or depression following surgery.

- **Return to Daily Activities:** Gradually reintroducing normal activities or sports without causing harm.

2. Stages of Post-Operative Rehabilitation

- **Acute Phase (0-2 weeks post-surgery):**

- Focus on pain control, reducing swelling, and gentle movement. Techniques like cold therapy, gentle passive movements, and isometric may be used.

- The patient may need to wear braces or use crutches.

- **Subacute Phase (2-6 weeks post-surgery):-**

- Introduction of active exercises to increase strength, balance, and mobility. Gradual return to weight-bearing activities if applicable.

- Continued physical therapy to restore range of motion.

- **Late Phase (6 weeks and beyond):-**

- Functional training becomes more intense, aiming to restore full strength, balance, and endurance.

- Progressive exercises to enhance mobility, depending on the type of surgery (e.g., hip, knee, shoulder).

- Focus on returning to work or sports-specific activities.

3. Types of Therapy in Post-Operative Rehab:-

- **Physical Therapy (PT):** Customized exercise plans to strengthen muscles, improve mobility, and enhance endurance.

- **Occupational Therapy (OT):** Focuses on helping patients regain the ability to perform daily tasks (dressing, eating, etc.).

- **Manual Therapy:** Includes techniques like massage or manipulation to improve movement and reduce pain.

- **Aquatic Therapy:** Exercising in water to reduce stress on joints and promote movement in a low-impact environment.

4. Duration of Post-Operative Rehabilitation:-

- **Minor surgeries**: Recovery may take 4-6 weeks with minimal physical therapy.

- **Major surgeries (e.g., joint replacement, spinal surgery)**: May require 3-6 months of rehabilitation.

5. Factors Affecting Rehabilitation:-

- **Age and Overall Health:** Older individuals or those with chronic conditions may have longer recovery periods.

- **Type of Surgery:** More complex surgeries may require extended rehabilitation.

- **Adherence to the Rehab Program:** Patient commitment to exercises and lifestyle modifications affects the outcome.

- **Support System:** Encouragement from family, friends, and healthcare professionals aids recovery.

6. Common Complications

• **Muscle Atrophy:** Lack of movement can lead to muscle weakening, requiring extensive rehabilitation.

• **Scar Tissue Formation:** Can limit movement, sometimes requiring specialized treatments.

• **Delayed Healing:** Due to poor blood flow or infections, impacting the rehabilitation timeline.

7. Role of Nutrition and Lifestyle

• **Diet:** A balanced diet rich in proteins, vitamins, and minerals supports healing and muscle regeneration.

• **Hydration:** Essential for tissue recovery and preventing complications like blood clots.

• **Smoking Cessation:** Smoking delays wound healing and increases the risk of complications.

• **Physical Activity:** Appropriate physical activity, even mild walking,promotes circulation and recovery.

D) ACL reconstruction:-

ACL (Anterior Cruciate Ligament) reconstruction is a surgical procedure used to replace a torn ACL, one of the major ligaments in the knee. The ACL is crucial for stabilizing the knee joint, especially during activities that involve sudden changes in direction or pivoting. When the ACL is torn, it doesn't heal on its own, and surgery is often required for those wanting to return to an active lifestyle or sports.

Steps in ACL Reconstruction:

1. Preparation:

• The patient is typically placed under general anesthesia.

• Arthroscopic tools are inserted into the knee joint for a minimally invasive approach.

2. Graft Harvest:

• A graft is harvested to replace the torn ACL. Common sources of the graft include:

▶ Patellar tendon (between the kneecap and tibia).

▶ Hamstring tendon.

▶ Quadriceps tendon.

Allograft (tissue from a cadaver**).**

3. Graft Placement:

• The surgeon cleans up any damaged tissue in the knee.

• Small tunnels are drilled into the femur and tibia, where the ACL attaches.

• The graft is threaded through these tunnels and anchored in place using screws or other fixation devices.

4. Final Adjustments:

◆   The surgeon adjusts the tension of the new ACL to ensure proper knee stability.

◆   The incision is closed, and the knee is bandaged.

Recovery and Rehabilitation:-

• **Initial Phase (1-2 weeks):** Focus on

• **Later Phase (6 weeks to 3 months):** Functional exercises are introduced, with a focus on balance and agility.

• **Return to Sport (6-12 months):** Depending on the individual's progress, return to sports can take around 6-12 months, with clearance from the surgeon and physical therapist.

Physical therapy is essential to regain full strength, flexibility, and function of the knee.

E) Hip/knee replacement:-

Hip or knee replacement, also known as arthroplasty, is a surgical procedure to replace a damaged hip or knee joint with an artificial one, often due to conditions like arthritis, injury, or degenerative joint diseases. Here's an overview of each procedure:

Hip Replacement:

- **Total Hip Replacement:** The damaged ball-and-socket components of the hip joint are replaced with artificial implants.

- **Indications:** Hip osteoarthritis, rheumatoid arthritis, avascular necrosis, fractures, or hip joint deformities.

- **Procedure:** The femoral head (ball of the thighbone) is replaced with a metal or ceramic ball, and the socket (acetabulum) is replaced with a prosthetic cup.

- **Recovery:** Patients typically stay in the hospital for 1-3 days, followed by physical therapy. Full recovery may take 3 to 6 months.

Knee Replacement:

- **Total Knee Replacement (TKR):** The entire knee joint is replaced with artificial components.

- **Partial Knee Replacement:** Only the damaged portion of the knee is replaced.

- **Indications:** Severe osteoarthritis, knee injuries, or deformities.

- **Procedure:** The damaged cartilage and bone are replaced with metal or plastic implants to create a new, smooth joint surface.

• Recovery: Hospital stay of 2-3 days, followed by physical therapy for a few

• Blood clots

• Implant loosening

• Joint stiffness

Benefits:

- Pain relief

- Improved mobility

- Enhanced quality of life

Both surgeries are highly effective, with many patients experiencing significant improvement in their quality of life.

F) Fracture recovery and physiotherapy's role:-

Fracture recovery involves several stages, and physiotherapy plays a crucial role in ensuring that the bone heals properly and that function is restored to the affected area. Here's a detailed look at the process:

1. Fracture Healing Process:

Inflammatory Phase (First few days):

The body forms a blood clot (hematoma) at the fracture site, and inflammatory cells are sent to the area to begin the healing process.

Reparative Phase (Weeks): New bone (soft callus) begins to form around the fracture, which later hardens (hard callus) as the bone continues to heal.

Remodeling Phase (Months to Years): The bone strengthens and remodels itself to restore normal structure and function.

2. Physiotherapy's Role:

Early Stages (Imobilization /Initial Healing):

- **Goal:** Maintain muscle strength, circulation, and joint mobility around the injury site.

- **Techniques:**

- Gentle range of motion (ROM) exercises for joints above and below the fracture.

- Isometric exercises to maintain. muscle strength without moving the fractured area.

- Pain management techniques like ice, electrotherapy, or gentle soft tissue mobilization.

After Immobilization (Once the bone has begun healing):

- **Goal: Restore movement, strength, and function to the injured area.**

- **Techniques:**

- **ROM exercises:** Gradually increasing the range of movement in the affected joint.

- **Strengthening exercises:** Progressive resistance training for muscles weakened by immobilization.

- **Weight-bearing exercises (if appropriate):** Gradual loading of the affected bone to stimulate bone healing and strengthen the area.

- **Balance and proprioception exercises:** Help restore coordination and prevent future injury.

- **Gait training:** For leg fractures, physiotherapists guide patients in learning to walk again, often using aids like crutches or walkers initially.

Final Stages (Advanced Rehabilitation):

- **Goal:** Achieve full functional recovery and prevent long-term complications like stiffness or weakness.

- **Techniques:**

- **Functional training:** Exercises that mimic daily activities or sports to help patients return to normal activities.

- **Endurance training:** To improve overall fitness, especially after a long period of immobilization.

3. Benefits of Physiotherapy:

- **Prevent Muscle Atrophy:** Immobilization can cause muscle weakening, which physiotherapy helps prevent.

- **Maintain Joint Mobility:** Keeping nearby joints flexible prevents long-term stiffness.

- **Accelerate Healing:** Controlled movements can promote better circulation, speeding up the healing process.

- **Reduce Pain:** Gentle exercises and manual therapy can alleviate pain caused by stiffness or swelling. Prevent Re-injury: Strengthening and balance exercises help ensure the injured area is strong and stable before resuming full activities.

4. Timeframes:

the individual's progress.

G) Shoulder injuries (e.g., rotator cuff tears) :-

especially among athletes and individuals involved in physical labor. The shoulder is a highly mobile joint, making it susceptible to injury. Below is an overview of common types of shoulder injuries, their causes, symptoms, and treatment options.

1. Common Types of Shoulder Injuries:

a. Rotator Cuff Tear:

Description: The rotator cuff is a group of four muscles and tendons that stabilize the shoulder. Tears can occur from acute injury or degeneration over time.

- **Causes:** Repetitive overhead motions (e.g., throwing, lifting), trauma, or aging-related degeneration.

- **Symptoms:** Shoulder pain, weakness, limited range of motion, difficulty lifting the arm, or sleeping on the affected side.

- **Treatment:**

Rest, physical therapy, anti-inflammatory medications.

Severe cases may require surgical repair

b. Shoulder Dislocation:

- ✧ **Description:** When the upper arm bone (humerus) pops out of the shoulder socket (glenoid). Causes Trauma from falls, sports injuries, or accidents.

- ✧ **Symptoms:** Intense pain, visible deformity, swelling, and inability to move the shoulder,

- ✧ **Treatment:**

- Immediate reduction (realigning the bone) by a healthcare professional.

- Immobilization followed by physical therapy to restore mobility and strength.

- Recurrent dislocations may require surgery.

c. Shoulder Impingement:

- ✧ **Description:** When the rotator cuff tendons become trapped and compressed during shoulder movements, causing inflammation.

- ✧ **Causes:** Repetitive overhead activity, poor posture, or bone spurs.

- ✧ **Symptoms:** Pain with overhead movement , difficulty reaching behind the back, weakness, and tenderness.

- ✧ **Treatment:**

- Rest, physical therapy to improve posture and strengthen the shoulder.

- Anti-inflammatory medications or corticosteroid injections.

- Surgery may be needed in severe cases.

d. Labral Tear:

- ✧ **Description:** A tear in the cartilage (labrum) that lines the shoulder socket, which can destabilize the shoulder.

- ✧ **Causes:** Trauma, repetitive overhead motions, or sudden pulling. clicking or catching sensation, Symptoms: Deep shoulder pain, a weakness, and instability.

- ✧ **Treatment:**

- Rest, physical therapy to strengthen the shoulder muscles.

- Surgery may be required to repair the torn labrum.

e. Frozen Shoulder (Adhesive Capsulitis):

- ✧ **Description**: A condition where the shoulder becomes stiff and painful, leading to restricted movement.

- ✧ **Causes:** The exact cause is often unclear, but it can be associated with injury, surgery, or conditions like diabetes.

- ✧ **Symptoms:** Gradual onset of pain and stiffness, leading to a loss of shoulder movement.

- ✧ **Treatment:**

- ✧ Physical therapy to stretch and mobilize the joint.

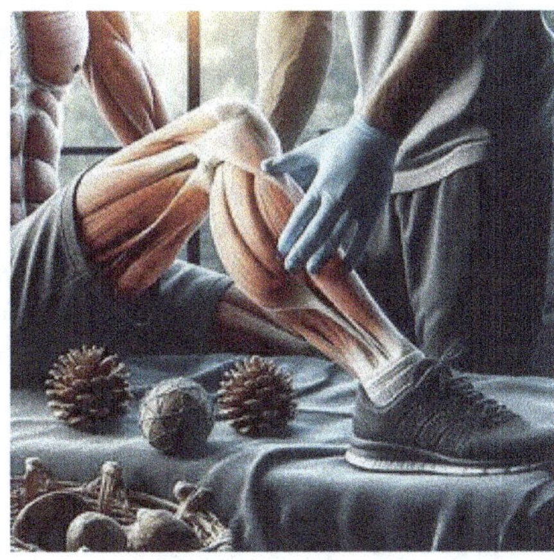

- ✧ Anti-inflammatory medications or corticosteroid injections.
- ✧ Rarely, surgery or manipulation under anesthesia may be necessary to improve mobility
- ✧ **f. Bursitis:**
- ✧ **Description:** Inflammation of the bursa, a small sac of fluid that cushions the shoulder joint.

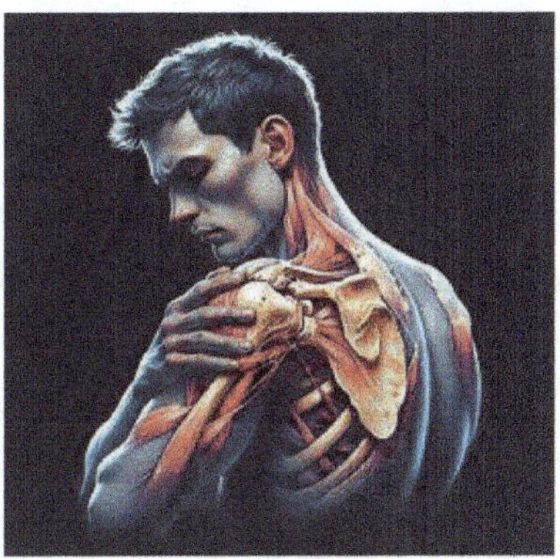

- ✧ **Causes:** Repetitive motion, injury, or prolonged pressure on the shoulder. Symptoms: Swelling, tenderness, and pain, especially when moving the shoulder or lying on it.
- ✧ **Treatment:**

• Rest, ice, and anti-inflammatory medications.

• Physical therapy to improve posture and strengthen surrounding muscles.

• In severe cases, corticosteroid injections or surgery to remove the inflamed bursa may be needed.

2. Diagnosis:

• **Physical Examination:** A healthcare professional will assess your range of

motion, strength, and the location of pain.

• **Imaging:** X-rays, MRI, or ultrasound.

may be used to diagnose the extent of the injury (e.g., torn rotator cuff dislocation).

• **Special Tests:** Specific movements or tests may be performed to identify shoulder instability or impingement.

3. Treatment Options:

• Rest and Activity Modification:

Reducing activities that aggravate the shoulder can help prevent further injury.

• Physical Therapy: A critical part of recovery, therapy focuses on restoring mobility, flexibility, and strength.

• Medications: Nonsteroidal anti-inflammatory drugs (NSAIDs) or corticosteroids to reduce pain and inflammation.

• Injections: Corticosteroid or platelet-rich plasma (PRP) injections may be used to decrease inflammation and promote healing.

• Surgery

Arthroscopic surgery for rotator cuff tears, labral tears, or shoulder impingement.

Open surgery for severe injuries like dislocations or fractures.

Joint replacement (arthroplasty)may be needed in severe degenerative cases.

4. Rehabilitation:

• Strengthening: Focused on rotator cuff muscles and shoulder stabilizers.

• Range of Motion: Stretching exercises to maintain and improve flexibility.

• Functional Training: Exercises that mimic daily activities or sports-related movements.

5. Prevention:

• Proper Warm-up: Always warm up before engaging in physical activity.

• Avoid Repetitive Overhead Movements: Take breaks during activities that involve repetitive overhead motions to prevent overuse injuries.

In conclusion, shoulder injuries can vary in severity, from mild inflammation to severe tears or dislocations. Early diagnosis and treatment, along with physiotherapy, play a critical role in full. recovery and restoring shoulder function.

6. Physiotherapy Techniques and Modalities:-

A)Manual therapy techniques :-

Manual therapy techniques are hands-on treatments that involve manipulating the muscles, joints, and soft tissues to reduce pain, improve mobility, and restore function. These techniques are commonly used in physical therapy, chiropractic care, and osteopathy. Some of the most common manual therapy techniques include:

1. **Soft Tissue Mobilization (STM):** This involves massaging muscles, tendons, and ligaments to release tension, break up scar tissue, and increase blood flow. It's effective for reducing muscle stiffness and pain.

2. Joint Mobilization: This technique uses controlled, passive movements to the joints to improve range of motion and decrease stiffness. The movements are usually slow and gentle, targeting specific joint dysfunctions.

3. Joint Manipulation (Thrust Technique): A high-velocity, low-amplitude thrust is applied to a joint to restore movement and alignment. This technique is often associated with chiropractic adjustments and can provide quick relief for certain types of joint pain.

4. Myofascial Release (MFR): This involves applying sustained pressure to the fascial tissue (connective tissue surrounding muscles) to release tightness and improve movement. It's helpful for treating chronic pain and mobility restrictions.

5. Muscle Energy Technique (MET): The therapist uses the patient's own muscle contractions against a controlled resistance to stretch tight muscles and mobilize joints. It's often used to treat muscle imbalances and joint restrictions.

6. Strain-Counterstrain: This is a gentle technique where the therapist positions the body in a way that shortens a painful muscle or joint, holding the position until the muscle relaxes and pain decreases.

7. Trigger Point Therapy: This technique focuses on applying pressure to specific points (trigger points) in the muscles that are painful and cause referred pain. Releasing these points can help alleviate muscle pain and tension.

8. Craniosacral Therapy: A gentle technique that focuses on the skull, spine, and sacrum to relieve tension in the central nervous system and promote overall well-being. It's often used for headaches, migraines, and stress-related issues.

9. Passive Range of Motion (PROM): The therapist moves the patient's joints through their range of motion without the patient's active involvement. This helps in improving flexibility and reducing stiffness, especially post-surgery or injury.

 (e.g., joint mobilization, soft tissue massage)

These techniques are often tailored to individual needs and conditions, aiming to promote healing and restore function.

B) Therapeutic exercises and stretches :-

Therapeutic exercises and stretches are crucial for improving flexibility, strength, and function, especially after injury or to manage conditions like arthritis, chronic pain, or muscle stiffness. Here are some commonly recommended exercises and stretches:

1. Range of Motion Exercises:-

• **Ankle Circles:** While seated or lying down, rotate your foot in circles, clockwise and counterclockwise. This helps with ankle flexibility and mobility.

• **Shoulder Rolls:** Gently roll your shoulders forward and backward to relieve tension and improve shoulder mobility.

• **Wrist Flexor Stretch:** Extend one arm straight in front of you with the palm facing up. Use the other hand to gently pull your fingers back toward your body.

2. Strengthening Exercises Clamshells (for hips): Lie on your side with your knees bent. Keep your feet together and lift the top knee as high as possible without moving your

- **pelvis. Bridges (for glutes and hamstrings):**

Lie on your back with your knees bent and feet flat on the floor. Lift your hips until your body forms a straight line from shoulders to knees.

- **Wall Push-Ups:** Stand a few feet away from a wall. Place your hands on the wall and do push-ups, maintaining a controlled pace. This is a gentler variation that strengthens arms and shoulders.

3. Stretching Exercises:-

- **Hamstring Stretch:** Sit on the floor with one leg extended. Reach toward your toes while keeping your back straight to stretch the back of your thigh.

- **Quadriceps Stretch:** Stand and grab your ankle behind you, pulling your heel toward your glutes while keeping your knees together.

- **Child's Pose (for lower back and shoulders):** Kneel on the floor, sit back on your heels, and reach your arms forward on the floor while lowering your chest toward the ground.

4. Core Stability Exercises:-

- **Pelvic Tilts:** Lie on your back with your knees bent. Tighten your stomach muscles and flatten your lower back against the floor, then release.

- **Bird Dog:** Start on your hands and knees. Extend one arm forward and the opposite leg back, keeping your back flat. Switch sides.

- **Plank:** Hold your body in a straight line, resting on your forearms and toes. Start with shorter holds, gradually increasing time.

5. Balance and Coordination:-

Single Leg Stance: Stand on one foot while holding onto a chair or counter for support. As you improve, try balancing without holding on.

- **Heel-to-Toe Walk:** Walk forward slowly, placing the heel of one foot directly in front of the toes of the other foot to improve coordination and balance.

6. Neck and Upper Back Stretches:-

- **Neck Side Stretch:** Sit or stand tall, and slowly bring your ear toward your shoulder to stretch the side of your neck.

- **Seated Spinal Twist:** Sit on a chair or the floor, twist your torso to one side, using your opposite arm to press against your knee or chair for a deeper stretch.

These exercises should be done gently, especially if you are recovering from an injury. Always consult a physical therapist or healthcare provider to ensure the exercises are suitable for your specific needs.

C) Electrotherapy (TENS, ultrasound therapy):-

Electrotherapy is the use of electrical energy as a medical treatment. It can be used for various purposes, including pain relief, muscle stimulation, tissue healing, and rehabilitation. There are several types of electrotherapy, each designed for specific conditions.

1. Transcutaneous Electrical Nerve Stimulation (TENS): A popular method for pain relief, TENS involves applying low-voltage electrical currents to the skin to stimulate nerves and block pain signals to the brain.

2. Electrical Muscle Stimulation (EMS): This method is used to stimulate muscle contractions, often in rehabilitation for patients who have lost muscle strength due to injury or surgery.

3. Interferential Therapy (IFT): This uses medium-frequency electrical currents to reduce pain and inflammation, often for deep tissue or joint injuries.

4. Galvanic Stimulation: This type of electrotherapy involves the use of direct current (DC) to stimulate blood flow, reduce swelling, and promote healing in injured tissues.

5. Iontophoresis: A method that uses electrical currents to deliver medication through the skin. It is often used to treat localized inflammation or pain.

6. Pulsed Shortwave Therapy (PSWT): This form of therapy applies high-frequency electromagnetic waves to reduce pain and inflammation and promote tissue repair.

7.Ultrasound Therapy:

Mechanism: Ultrasound therapy uses high-frequency sound waves that penetrate deep into tissues, generating heat and promoting healing at a cellular level. The sound waves cause soft tissues to vibrate, increasing blood flow and reducing inflammation.

Uses: It's commonly used to treat soft tissue injuries, muscle spasms, joint inflammation, and scar tissue. Conditions like tendonitis, bursitis, and ligament injuries respond well to ultrasound therapy.

Benefits: Accelerates tissue repair, reduces inflammation, and can break down scar tissue. It also helps in increasing the extensibility of tight muscles and ligaments.

Considerations: Ultrasound therapy should not be applied over bone fractures, near pacemakers, or over areas with malignant tumors.

Electrotherapy is widely used in physical therapy, sports rehabilitation, and pain management, but the appropriateness of its use depends on individual patient conditions and medical advice.

D) Hydrotherapy:-

Hydrotherapy, also known as water therapy, is the use of water in various forms (such as steam, liquid, or ice) for pain relief, physical therapy, and general wellness. It's been practiced for centuries in different cultures and can involve treatments like baths, showers, steam rooms, and specific exercises in water.

Some common forms of hydrotherapy include:

1. Hot and Cold Treatments: Alternating hot and cold water is believed to stimulate blood circulation and promote healing.

2. Water Exercises: Activities like swimming or water aerobics help relieve joint pressure, especially for those with arthritis or muscle injuries.

3. Bathing Therapies: Warm baths with added salts or essential oils can help relax muscles, improve circulation, and reduce stress.

4. Steam Rooms or Saunas: Exposure to steam is used to detoxify the skin, improve respiratory health, and increase circulation.

Hydrotherapy can be beneficial for conditions like arthritis, muscle pain, stress, and even certain respiratory or skin conditions. However, it should be done with guidance, especially for individuals with heart conditions or other chronic health issues.

E) Dry needling in physiotherapy:-

often used by physical therapists, chiropractors, and other healthcare professionals to treat musculoskeletal pain. It involves inserting thin, filiform needles into the skin and muscles at specific points, known as trigger points, to release muscle tightness, reduce pain, and improve range of motion.

The technique is called "dry" needling because, unlike injections, no substance is injected into the body. The needles stimulate the muscles, fascia, and connective tissues, promoting healing through mechanical stimulation. This can help alleviate issues such as chronic pain, tension headaches, and sports injuries.

Dry needling differs from acupuncture in its approach and philosophy, although both use needles. While acupuncture is rooted in traditional Chinese medicine and focuses on balancing energy flow or "Qi" along meridians, dry needling is based on modern Western anatomy and aims to target trigger points directly to alleviate pain and improve function.

Common conditions treated by dry needling include:

• Back and neck pain

• Muscle strains

• Joint pain

• Tendonitis

• Sports injuries

It can be particularly effective when combined with other physical therapy treatments like manual therapy, exercise, or stretching.

F) Use of heat and cold therapy:-

Heat and cold therapy are common treatments used to relieve pain, reduce inflammation, and improve healing for a variety of conditions. Each type of therapy has specific uses and benefits depending on the nature of the injury or ailment.

Heat Therapy (Thermotherapy):

Heat therapy is used to relax muscles, increase circulation, and promote healing by delivering warmth to the affected area.

Uses:-

Chronic Muscle Pain: Heat relaxes tense muscles and can help alleviate soreness or stiffness, often recommended for long-term conditions like arthritis, fibromyalgia, and back pain.

Joint Stiffness: Applying heat can improve the flexibility of joints, making it useful for osteoarthritis or conditions where joint movement is limited.

Stress Relief and Muscle Tension: Heat therapy is effective for reducing tension in muscles caused by stress or overuse.

Before Exercise: Applying heat before physical activity can loosen muscles and improve flexibility, reducing the risk of injury.

Methods:

- Hot packs or heating pads

- Warm baths or showers

- Steam towels

- Paraffin wax treatments

- Ultrasound therapy (for deep heating)

Cold Therapy (Cryotherapy):-

Cold therapy is used to reduce inflammation, swelling, and pain by numbing the affected area and constricting blood vessels, which limits blood flow.

Uses:

Acute Injuries: Ice is most effective immediately after a sprain, strain, or other acute injuries to reduce swelling and inflammation. This is part of the R.I.C.E (Rest, Ice, Compression, Elevation) method for treating acute injuries.

Bruising and Swelling: Cold therapy can limit blood flow to the area, preventing further tissue damage and reducing bruising and swelling.

Pain Relief: Ice can numb nerve endings and reduce pain, especially after an intense workout or overuse injury.

Post-Surgical Recovery: It is often used after surgeries to minimize swelling and pain in the affected areas.

Methods:

- Ice packs or gel packs

- Cold baths

- Cold compresses

- Cryotherapy machines (for targeted or whole-body cooling)

When to Use Each Therapy:

Cold Therapy: Best for acute injuries, inflammation, and swelling within the first 48 hours.

Heat Therapy: Ideal for chronic conditions, muscle tightness, or injuries that have already passed the acute stage.

When to Avoid:

- **Heat:** Should be avoided immediately after an acute injury (within the first 48 hours) as it may increase swelling.

- **Cold:** Should not be used on stiff muscles or joints that are not swollen, as it can make the muscles even tighter.

Both therapies can be part of a broader pain management or rehabilitation plan,depending on the injury or condition.

8. Home Exercises and Self-Care :-

A) Basic stretching routines for different body parts :-

1. Neck:

- **Neck Tilt:** Sit or stand. Gently tilt your head towards one shoulder, holding for 15-30 seconds. Repeat on the other side.

- **Neck Rotation**: Slowly rotate your head in a circle, moving it side to side, forward, and backward. Do 5 rotations in each direction.

2. Shoulders:

- **Shoulder Roll:** Roll your shoulders forward in a circular motion 10 times, then roll them backward 10 times.

- **Cross-Body Shoulder Stretch**: Bring one arm across your body and hold it with the other arm for 15-30 seconds. Switch arms.

3. Chest:

- **Chest Opener Stretch:** Stand with your hands clasped behind your back. Lift your chest and pull your shoulders back. Hold for 20-30 seconds.

4. Upper Back:

- **Cat-Cow Stretch:** On all fours, arch your back upward (like a cat) and hold for a few seconds, then dip your back downward (cow position) and hold. Repeat 10 times.

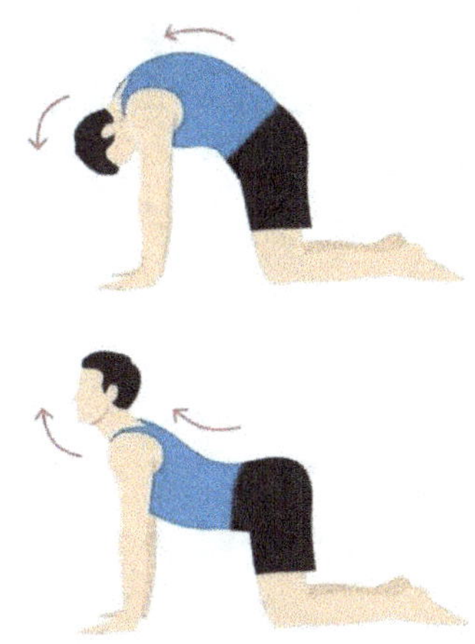

5. Lower Back:

• **Child's Pose**: Kneel on the floor, then sit back on your heels and stretch your arms forward, lowering your chest towards the floor. Hold for 30 seconds.

• **Seated Forward Fold:** Sit on the floor with legs extended straight. Reach forward toward your toes, holding for 20-30 seconds.

6. Hips:

• **Hip Flexor Stretch:** Kneel on one knee with the other leg in front, foot flat on the floor. Push your hips forward gently, feeling a stretch in the hip of the back leg. Hold for 20-30 seconds, then switch legs.

7. Hamstrings:

• **Standing Hamstring Stretch:** Stand and place one foot on a bench or raised surface. Keep your leg straight and hinge at your hips to lean forward. Hold for 20-30 seconds, then switch legs.

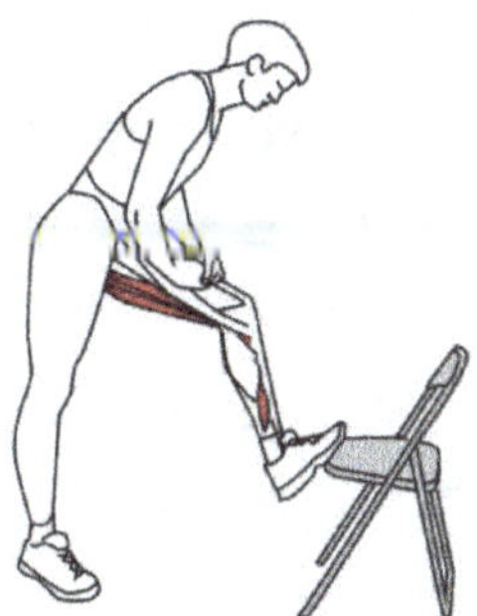

8. Quadriceps:

• **Standing Quad Stretch**: Stand on one leg, pulling the other foot toward your glutes, holding your ankle. Hold for 20-30 seconds, then switch legs.

9. Calves:

• **Standing Calf Stretch:** Stand with one leg behind the other. Keep the back leg straight with the heel on the ground and bend the front knee. Hold for 20-30 seconds, then switch sides.

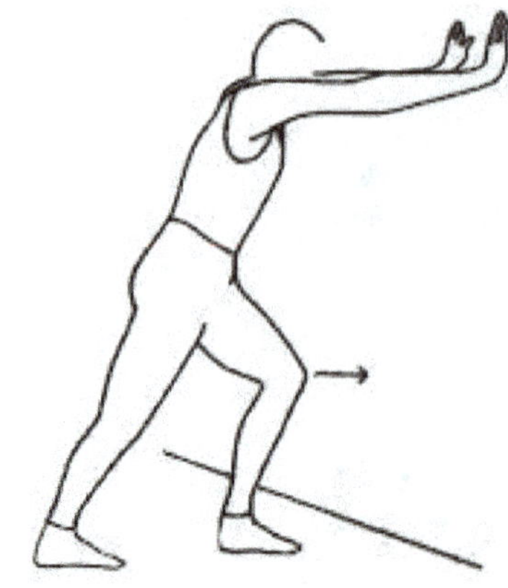

Standing calf stretch

10. Ankles:

• **Ankle Circles:** While sitting or standing, lift one foot off the ground and rotate the ankle in circles 10 times in each direction. Switch feet.

Repeat this routine 1-2 times, aiming to hold each stretch gently without bouncing.

 This helps improve flexibility and prevent injuries.

B) Core strengthening exercises for stability:-

Core strengthening exercises are great for improving stability, balance, and overall body strength. Here are some effective exercises to target your core muscles:

1. Plank

• **How to do it: Start in a push-up position with your forearms on the ground. Keep your body in a straight line from your head to your heels, engaging your core.**

• **Benefits:** Strengthens the entire core and improves posture and stability.

• **Duration:** Hold for 20-60 seconds.

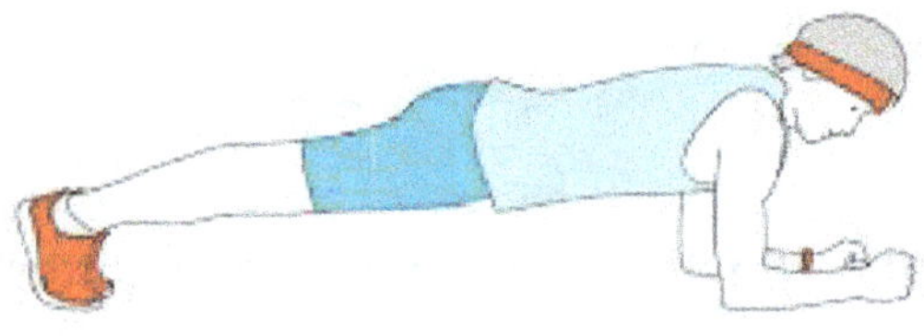

2. Dead Bug

• **How to do it:** Lie on your back with arms extended toward the ceiling and knees bent at 90 degrees. Slowly lower your right arm and left leg toward the floor, then return to the starting position and switch sides.

- **Benefits:** Improves core stability and coordination.

Reps: 10-12 reps per side.

3. Bird-Dog

How to do it: Start on your hands and knees. Extend your right arm and left leg simultaneously, keeping your back flat and core engaged. Return to the starting position and switch sides.

- **Benefits:** Enhances balance, stability, and core strength.
- **Reps:** 10-12 reps per side.

4. Russian Twists

- **How to do it:** Sit on the floor with your knees bent and feet off the ground. Lean back slightly and rotate your torso to one side, then the other, while holding a weight or medicine ball.

Benefits: Targets obliques and improves rotational stability.

Reps: 15-20 reps per side.

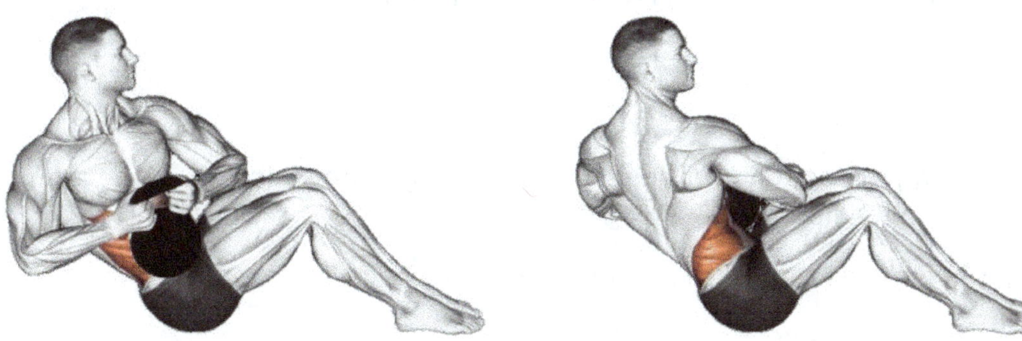

5. Leg Raises

- **How to do it:** Lie on your back with your legs extended. Lift your legs until they are perpendicular to the floor, then slowly lower them back down without letting them touch the ground.

Benefits: Strengthens the lower abdominals.

- **Reps:** 10-15 reps.

6. Side Plank

- **How to do it:** Lie on your side with one forearm on the ground and your body. in a straight line. Lift your hips off the ground and hold the position while engaging your core.
- **Benefits:** Strengthens the obliques and improves lateral stability.
- **Duration:** Hold for 20-45 seconds per side.

7. Glute Bridge

- **How to do it:** Lie on your back with knees bent and feet flat on the ground. Lift your hips toward the ceiling while squeezing your glutes, then slowly lower back down.

• **Benefits:** Strengthens the core and glutes, improving overall stability.

Reps: 12-15 reps.

Incorporating these exercises into your routine 2-3 times a week can help improve your core strength and stability over time.

C) Exercises for posture correction:-

Improving posture is essential for reducing discomfort and preventing long-term issues. Here are some effective exercises that can help correct posture by strengthening the muscles that support proper alignment:

1. Cat-Cow Stretch

• **How to do it:** Start on your hands and knees in a tabletop position. Inhale as you arch your back (cow pose), lifting your head and tailbone. Exhale as you round your back (cat pose), tucking your chin and pelvis.

Benefits: Increases flexibility of the spine and helps release tension in the back.

Reps: 10-15 cycles.

2. Child's Pose:-

How to do it: Kneel on the floor, sit back on your heels, and stretch your arms forward on the ground while lowering your forehead to the floor.

Benefits: Stretches the back, shoulders, and neck; promotes relaxation.

Duration: Hold for 30 seconds to 1 minute.

3. Wall Angels:-

• **How to do it:** Stand with your back against a wall, feet a few inches away from the wall. Keep your arms bent at 90 degrees and pressed against the wall. Slowly raise your arms overhead while maintaining contact with the wall.

Benefits: Strengthens upper back muscles and improves shoulder mobility.

• **Reps:** 10-12 reps.

4. Thoracic Extension

How to do it: Sit or stand with a tall spine. Place your hands behind your head and gently arch your upper back while pulling your elbows back.

Benefits: Opens up the chest and improves thoracic spine mobility.

Reps: 10-12 reps.

5. Chest Opener Stretch:-

How to do it: Stand tall and interlace your fingers behind your back. Straighten your arms and gently lift them while opening your chest.

Benefits: Stretches the chest and strengthens the upper back.

Duration: Hold for 20-30 seconds.

6. Shoulder Blade Squeeze:-

• **How to do it:-** Sit or stand with your arms at your sides. Squeeze your shoulder blades together as if pinching a pencil between them.

Benefits: Strengthens the muscles between the shoulder blades and improves upper back posture.

Reps: 10-15 reps.

7. Plank with Shoulder Taps:-

How to do it: Start in a plank position. While maintaining a stable core, lift one hand to tap the opposite shoulder, alternating sides.

Benefits: Strengthens the core and shoulders while promoting stability.

• **Reps**: 10-12 taps per side.

8. Hip Flexor Stretch:-

How to do it: Kneel on one knee with the other foot in front, creating a 90-degree angle. Push your hips forward while keeping your back straight.

Benefits: Stretches tight hip flexors, which can contribute to poor posture.

 Duration: Hold for 20-30 seconds per side.

9. Glute Bridge:-

How to do it: Lie on your back with knees bent and feet flat. Lift your hips while squeezing your glutes, keeping your shoulders on the ground. Benefits: Strengthens the glutes and lower back, helping to maintain proper pelvic alignment.

• **Reps:** 12-15 reps.

• **How to do it:** Use resistance bands or a cable machine. Sit or stand, pulling the band/machine handle towards your torso while keeping your elbows.

10. Seated Row:-

close to your body. Benefits: Strengthens the upper back and rear shoulders, counteracting slumped shoulders.

Reps: 10-15 reps.

Incorporate these exercises into your routine 2-3 times a week, focusing on maintaining proper form. This will help improve your posture over time and reduce discomfort.

D) Injury prevention strategies through exercise:-

Injury prevention strategies through exercise focus on enhancing physical fitness, improving body mechanics, and reducing the risk of injuries during physical activities or sports. Here are some effective strategies:

1. Warm-Up and Cool-Down:-

Warm-Up: Begin with dynamic stretching and low-intensity movements to increase blood flow and flexibility. This prepares muscles and joints for more strenuous activity.

Cool-Down: Follow with static stretching after exercise to promote flexibility and aid recovery.

2. Strength Training:-

Engage in a balanced strength training program that targets major muscle groups. Strong muscles help support joints and reduce the risk of injuries. Focus on:

- Core stability

- Functional movements

- Weight-bearing exercises

3. Flexibility and Mobility Work:-

Incorporate regular stretching routines, yoga, or Pilates to enhance flexibility and mobility. This can help prevent injuries by improving range of motion and joint health.

4. Balance and Coordination Exercises:-

Include exercises that improve balance and coordination, such as:

- Single-leg stands

- Balance boards

- Agility drills

These exercises enhance proprioception, reducing the risk of falls and related injuries.

5. Sport-Specific Training:-

- Tailor exercise programs to the specific demands of the sport or activity. This may include:

- Agility drills for sports like soccer or basketball

- Plyometric training for activities requiring explosive movements

6. Gradual Progression:-

Increase the intensity, duration, and frequency of workouts gradually. Sudden changes in activity levels can lead to overuse injuries. Follow the "10% rule" (increase volume or intensity by no more than 10% per week).

7. Cross-Training:-

- Engage in various forms of exercise to prevent overuse injuries. Cross-training allows different muscle groups to rest while still maintaining overall fitness.

8. Proper Footwear and Equipment:-

- Use appropriate footwear that provides support and cushioning. Ensure any sports equipment is well-maintained and suitable for your body type and activity.

9. Hydration and Nutrition:-

• Maintain adequate hydration and a balanced diet to support overall health and recovery. Dehydration and poor nutrition can increase injury risk.

10. Listen to Your Body:-

• Pay attention to signs of fatigue or pain. Rest and modify activities as necessary to prevent injury. Implement recovery strategies like foam rolling or massage.

11. Education and Training:

• Consider workshops or training sessions on injury prevention techniques specific to your sport or activity. Understanding proper techniques can reduce the likelihood of injury.

12. Regular Health Check-Ups:

• Regular physical assessments can help identify potential risk factors or imbalances, allowing for early intervention.

Implementing these strategies can significantly reduce the risk of injuries and promote long-term physical health and performance.

E) Guidelines on ergonomics and correct posture at home and work:-

 Here are some guidelines on ergonomics and correct posture for both home and work environments:

General Ergonomic Principles:

1. Neutral Posture: Maintain a neutral body position where joints are aligned and relaxed. This reduces strain and discomfort.

2. Support: Use furniture that supports your body's natural curves. Chairs should have lumbar support, and desks should be at a height that keeps your elbows at 90 degrees.

3. Movement: Regularly change your position and take breaks to move around to avoid prolonged static postures.

Ergonomics at a Desk:

1. Chair Height: Adjust your chair so your feet rest flat on the floor and your knees are at or slightly below hip level.

2. Screen Position: Position your monitor at eye level, about an arm's length away. The top of the screen should be at or slightly below eye level.

3. Keyboard and Mouse: Keep your keyboard and mouse close enough so you can use them without stretching. Your wrists should be straight, and hands should float above the keyboard.

4. Document Placement: If you use documents, place them close to the monitor to avoid neck strain.

Sitting Posture:

1. Feet: Keep your feet flat on the floor or on a footrest.

2. Back: Sit all the way back in your chair with your lower back supported.

3. Shoulders: Keep your shoulders relaxed and avoid hunching them.

Standing Workstations:

1. Height Adjustment: Ensure your workstation allows for proper arm position with elbows at 90 degrees.

2. Foot Position: Shift your weight from one foot to the other, or use a footrest to alternate foot positioning.

3. Monitor Height: Similar to sitting, ensure the monitor is at eye level.

Home Office Setup

1. Lighting: Ensure adequate lighting to reduce eye strain; avoid glare on screens.

2. Organization: Keep frequently used items within reach to avoid excessive stretching.

3. Breaks: Schedule regular breaks (5-10 minutes every hour) to stand, stretch, or walk around.

Additional Tips:-

Exercise: Incorporate exercises and stretches into your routine to strengthen your back and core muscles.

Hydration: Stay hydrated to maintain overall health and help with concentration.

Footwear: Wear supportive shoes, especially if you are standing for long periods.

Stretching and Movement:-

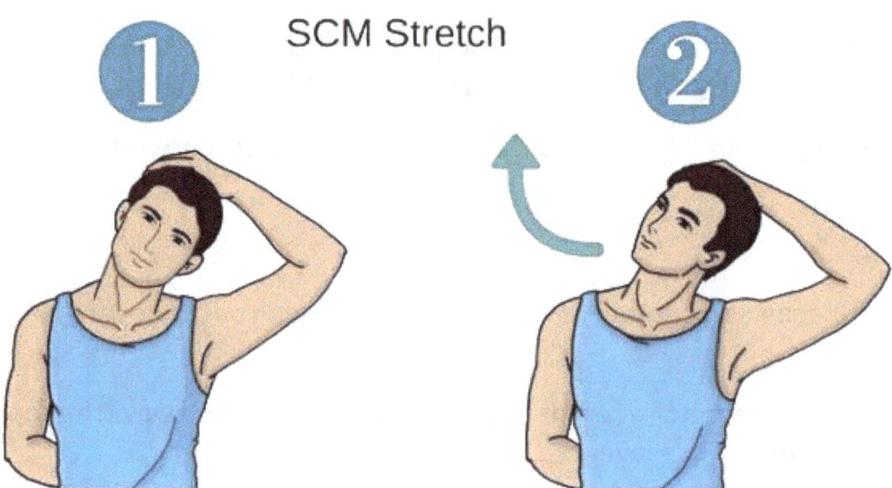

1. Neck Stretches: Gently tilt your head to one side and hold for a few seconds, then switch sides.

2. Shoulder Rolls: Roll your shoulders forward and backward to relieve tension.

3. Wrist and Finger Stretches: Extend and flex your wrists and fingers to prevent strain.

Following these ergonomic principles can help reduce discomfort and the risk of injury, leading to a healthier and more productive work environment.

8. Physiotherapy for Special Populations:-

A)Physiotherapy during pregnancy (prenatal and postnatal care):

Physiotherapy during pregnancy can play a crucial role in promoting physical health and comfort for expectant mothers. Here are some key points regarding its benefits, techniques, and considerations:

Benefits of Physiotherapy during Pregnancy:

1. Pain Relief: Physiotherapy can help alleviate common pregnancy-related discomforts, such as back pain, pelvic pain, and sciatica.

2. Improved Mobility: Tailored exercises can enhance flexibility and strength, which can ease daily activities and improve overall mobility.

3. Posture Correction: Physiotherapists can provide guidance on maintaining proper posture, which can reduce strain on the spine and muscles.

4. Breathing Techniques: Learning effective breathing techniques can help during labor and delivery.

5. Preparation for Labor: Specific exercises can strengthen the pelvic floor, improving support for the uterus and aiding in labor.

6. Mental Well-being: Physical activity and therapy can also contribute to reduced anxiety and improved mood during pregnancy.

Physiotherapy Techniques:

• **Exercise Therapy:** Customized exercise programs focusing on strength, flexibility, and endurance. Common exercises include pelvic tilts, stretching, and low-impact aerobic activities.

Manual Therapy: Techniques such as massage and joint mobilization can help relieve tension and improve joint function.

Education: Providing information on body mechanics, posture, and strategies for coping with discomfort.

• **Hydrotherapy:** Water exercises can be particularly beneficial, as they reduce stress on the joints and provide a gentle way to stay active.

Considerations:

• **Consultation:** It's essential to consult a healthcare provider before starting any physiotherapy program during pregnancy, especially if there are existing medical conditions or complications.

Qualified Therapist: Ensure that the physiotherapist has experience working with pregnant women and is knowledgeable about pregnancy-related issues.

on your back after the first trimester.

- Stay hydrated and avoid overheating during exercise.

- Listen to your body and stop if you experience pain, dizziness, or shortness of breath.

Incorporating physiotherapy into a pregnancy wellness routine can support both physical and emotional health, leading to a more comfortable experience.

B) Physiotherapy for children with developmental disorders:

Physiotherapy for children with developmental disorders focuses on improving mobility, posture, strength, and motor skills. It helps children with conditions such as cerebral palsy, Down syndrome, autism spectrum disorder (ASD), and developmental coordination disorder to reach their developmental milestones and function more independently.

Key aspects of physiotherapy for children with developmental disorders include:

1. Early Intervention: Early diagnosis and intervention can significantly improve outcomes. Physiotherapy aims to stimulate normal motor development and prevent secondary complications like contractures or joint deformities.

2. Individualized Therapy Plans: Each child's therapy plan is tailored to their specific needs, including assessments of muscle tone, balance, coordination, and range of motion.

3. Gross Motor Skills Development: Physiotherapists work on improving fundamental movements like sitting, crawling, walking, and running. These skills are critical for independence and daily activities.

4. Strengthening and Flexibility: Therapy may involve exercises and activities designed to strengthen muscles, improve flexibility, and enhance posture, especially in children with weak or stiff muscles.

5. Balance and Coordination: Improving balance and coordination helps children participate in play and sports, boosts confidence, and reduces the risk of falls.

6. Use of Adaptive Equipment: Sometimes, children may need support through equipment like walkers, braces, or special footwear. Physiotherapists assist in selecting and training the child to use such aids.

7. Parental Involvement: Parents play a critical role in the physiotherapy process. Physiotherapists often guide parents on how to assist with exercises and incorporate therapy into daily routines.

8. Therapies in Various Settings: Physiotherapy may occur in clinics, schools, or homes, depending on the child's needs and convenience. Therapy in natural environments often promotes functional and social learning.

9. Multidisciplinary Approach: Collaboration with other professionals such as occupational therapists, speech therapists, and doctors is common to ensure a holistic approach to the child's development.

Physiotherapy helps improve the quality of life for children with developmental disorders by supporting their physical abilities, promoting independence, and encouraging participation in daily activities and social interactions.

C) Geriatric care and fall prevention :

Geriatric care, especially in the context of fall prevention, is crucial for enhancing the quality of life and maintaining the independence of older adults. Falls are a leading cause of injury among older people, and preventing them is a key goal in geriatric care.

prevention:

Here's an overview of important aspects of geriatric care related to fall

1. Risk Factors for Falls in Older Adults:

• **Muscle Weakness and Poor Balance:** As people age, they may lose muscle strength, leading to difficulty maintaining balance.

• **Vision Problems:** Age-related conditions like cataracts or glaucoma can impair vision, increasing the risk of tripping or falling.

Chronic Conditions: Conditions such as arthritis, osteoporosis, heart disease, and neurological disorders (like Parkinson's disease) can increase fall risk.

• **Medications:** Some medications, especially those that cause dizziness or drowsiness (e.g., sedatives, blood pressure drugs), may contribute to falls.

• **Home Hazards:** Clutter, slippery floors, inadequate lighting, and loose rugs or carpets are common hazards.

• **Cognitive Decline:** Memory problems or confusion, as seen in dementia, can lead to poor judgment or missteps, increasing fall risk.

2. Strategies for Fall Prevention:

Strengthening and Balance

• **Exercises:** Physical therapy programs focused on building muscle strength and improving balance (e.g., tai chi, walking programs) are highly effective in fall prevention.

• **Environmental Modifications:** Simple changes like removing tripping hazards (loose rugs, cords), installing grab bars in bathrooms, and improving lighting can drastically reduce fall risks at home.

• **Use of Assistive Devices:** Canes, walkers, and other mobility aids can help maintain balance and reduce the likelihood of falls. It's important that these devices are properly fitted by a healthcare professional.

• **Medication Review:** Regular reviews of medications by healthcare providers can help identify and reduce the use of drugs that contribute to fall risk.

- **Footwear Choices:** Non-slip, well-fitted shoes can help prevent falls. Older adults should avoid high heels, loose slippers, or shoes with poor support.

- **Vision and Hearing Checks:** Regular check-ups to ensure optimal vision and hearing are important, as impaired senses can lead to falls.

3. Multidisciplinary Approach:

- **Healthcare Team Involvement:** Physicians, geriatric specialists, physiotherapists, occupational therapists, and nutritionists all work together to ensure comprehensive fall prevention.

- **Family and Caregiver Support:** Family members and caregivers play a vital role in helping older adults with daily activities, monitoring for fall hazards, and encouraging safe habits.

4. Exercise Programs for Fall Prevention:

- Programs specifically designed for older adults can focus on improving flexibility, strength, and balance. Activities like yoga, Pilates, and water-based exercises are gentle yet effective.

5. Assistive Technologies:

- **Fall Detection Devices:** Wearable devices and home systems that detect falls can alert caregivers or medical professionals immediately after a fall, providing timely help.

- **Home Monitoring Systems:** Smart home systems can monitor movement and detect potential risks. or changes in behavior that might signal a fall risk.

6. Addressing Nutritional Deficiencies:

- **Bone Health**: Ensuring adequate intake of calcium and vitamin D is critical for bone strength, reducing the risk of fractures if a fall occurs.

- **Hydration:** Dehydration can cause dizziness or weakness, increasing the chance of falling.

Rehabilitation:

After a fall, rehabilitation is essential for regaining mobility and preventing future falls. Physiotherapy and occupational therapy help restore strength and function. Psychological Support: A fall can cause a fear of falling again, leading to reduced activity and isolation. Counseling and support groups may help older adults regain confidence.

By combining these strategies, geriatric care professionals aim to minimize fall risks, enhance mobility, and help older adults maintain independence and a higher quality of life.

D) Physiotherapy for athletes:

Physiotherapy for athletes is essential for optimizing performance, preventing injuries, and aiding recovery. It involves various techniques to address sports-specific demands on the body.

1. Injury Prevention

- **Functional assessments:**

Physiotherapists assess an athlete's movement patterns to identify potential risk factors for injury, such as muscle imbalances or joint instability.

Strengthening programs: Tailored exercises focus on strengthening muscles, improving flexibility, and enhancing endurance to reduce injury risk.

Neuromuscular training: This improves coordination, balance, and agility, which are crucial for preventing injuries during high-performance activities.

2. Rehabilitation

Acute Injury Management:

Physiotherapists treat sprains, strains, ligament tears, and fractures through manual therapy, exercises, and modalities like ultrasound or cryotherapy.

Post-surgical rehab: After surgeries like ACL reconstruction or rotator cuff repair, physiotherapy is vital for regaining strength, mobility, and function.

Progressive loading: Exercises are progressively adjusted to restore the athlete's full capacity while ensuring the healing process is respected.

3. Performance Enhancement

Flexibility and Mobility: Techniques like dynamic stretching, joint mobilization, and soft tissue therapy ensure optimal flexibility and range of motion.

Strength and Conditioning:

Customized strength programs help improve power, speed, and endurance specific to an athlete's sport.

Biomechanical analysis:

Physiotherapists analyze running, jumping, or throwing techniques to improve efficiency and reduce stress on muscles and joints.

4.Recovery

Massage Therapy: Helps reduce muscle soreness, improve circulation, and promote faster recovery after intense workouts or competition.

Cryotherapy and Hydrotherapy: These methods help reduce inflammation and aid in quicker recovery from strenuous physical activity.

• **Stretching and Myofascial Release:** Techniques to relieve muscle tightness and maintain flexibility post-exercise.

5. Sports-Specific Training:

• Physiotherapists design programs that mimic the specific physical demands of the sport, enhancing performance while focusing on injury resilience.

• Overall, physiotherapy plays a crucial role in an athlete's career by maintaining optimal health and performance. It ensures that athletes can safely push their limits and recover effectively from injuries.

E) Working with patients with chronic pain

Working with parents who have chronic pain requires a sensitive and compassionate approach. Chronic pain can significantly affect their emotional, mental, and physical well-being, often impacting their ability to engage in parenting activities. Here are some key strategies for supporting parents in this situation:

(e.g., fibromyalgia)

1. Understanding Their Condition:

• Learn about the specific chronic pain condition the parent is experiencing to better understand their limitations and challenges.

• Show empathy towards their pain, validating their experience and recognizing that chronic pain is real, even if it's invisible.

2. Encouraging Open Communication:

• Encourage parents to talk openly with their children about their pain in age-appropriate ways. This helps children understand why their parent may be less physically active or why they need rest.

• Open communication with the co-parent or other family members is also crucial to distribute responsibilities effectively.

3. Fostering Coping Skills:

• Help parents develop coping strategies, such as relaxation techniques, mindfulness, or pacing their activities. These can make managing daily life easier.

• Parents can also model healthy coping mechanisms for their children, teaching them resilience and problem-solving.

4. Adapting Parenting Tasks:

• Offer tips on adjusting parenting tasks to be less physically demanding. For example, finding ways to sit while playing with children, or creating a routine that allows for rest periods.

• Adaptive equipment or modifications in the home environment (such as low shelves, using assistive devices) can help manage tasks more easily.

5. Supporting Mental Health:

• Chronic pain can lead to mental health challenges, such as depression or anxiety. Encourage parents to seek mental health support if needed. Therapy or support groups may be beneficial.

• Encourage self-care practices and routines that prioritize their emotional and physical well-being.

6. Encouraging Family Support:

• Building a network of family or friends who can help with childcare or household tasks when needed is critical. It alleviates some of the pressure on the parent.

• Encourage parents to ask for help when they need it, and educate children about how they can assist in manageable ways.

7. Co-Parenting and Partnership:

• If there is a co-parent, ensure there's a clear distribution of responsibilities, allowing the parent with chronic pain to rest when necessary.

• Encourage discussions about parenting roles to ensure the parent with pain doesn't feel like they're falling short.

8. Recognizing Emotional Impact on Children:

Chronic pain can affect the parent-child dynamic, and children may feel worried or anxious about their parent's condition. Parents may need support in addressing these concerns with their children. Helping children express their feelings through conversation, art, or play can be a good way to manage these emotions.

9. Incorporating Physical Therapy:

• If appropriate, encourage the parent to engage in physical therapy or gentle movement practices, such as yoga or stretching, that might ease their pain and improve their mobility, which can help with parenting activities.

10. Providing Resources:

Recommend local or online support groups, educational materials about chronic pain, or services for respite care to ease some of the burdens on the family.

9. Case Studies:-

A) Case study 1: Physiotherapy for chronic back pain:-

Background:

Patient: Mr. J, 45-year-old male

Occupation: Office worker, spends 8-10 hours sitting

Chief complaint: Chronic lower back pain for the past two years, exacerbated by prolonged sitting and certain physical activities

Previous treatment: Medications (NSAIDs), intermittent physical therapy. occasional chiropractic adjustments

Medical history: Mild scoliosis, occasional muscle spasms, no prior surgeries **Physical activity level:** Sedentary due to pain

Goals: Reduce pain, improve mobility, and regain normal function for daily activities

Initial Evaluation:

Subjective Assessment:

• **Pain location:** Localized in the lumbar region (L4-L5)

• **Pain intensity:** 5-7/10 on a Visual Analog Scale (VAS)

• **Aggravating factors:** Prolonged sitting, bending forward, and lifting heavy objects

•**Relieving factors:** Lying down, heat therapy

• **Sleep disturbance:** Poor sleep due to pain when turning in bed

Objective Assessment:

•**Posture:** Mild forward head posture, slouched sitting posture Range of motion: Limited flexion and extension of the lumbar spine

• **Muscle tightness:** Tightness in the hamstrings and lower back extensors Strength deficits: Weakness in core muscles, particularly the transversus abdominis and glutes

• **Neurological signs:** No evidence of radiculopathy or nerve compression (negative straight-leg raise test)

Physiotherapy Treatment Plan:

1. Education:

• Provided information on posture correction and ergonomic setup for work (adjusting chair, desk height, frequent breaks). Educated about the importance of staying active and avoiding prolonged sitting.

2. Manual Therapy:

• Soft tissue mobilization to reduce tension in the lower back muscles.

•Gentle joint mobilizations to improve lumbar spine mobility.

3. Exercise Program:

Phase 1 (Acute Phase Pain Control):

►Core stabilization exercises (e.g., pelvic tilts, drawing-in maneuvers).

►Isometric exercises to strengthen the deep core muscles without aggravating the pain.

►Gentle stretching of the hamstrings, hip flexors, and lumbar spine to improve flexibility.

Phase 2 (Subacute Phase - Strengthening and Mobility):

► Progress to dynamic core exercises (e.g., bird dog, bridges) to improve strength and endurance.

►Introduction of controlled spinal movements (e.g., cat-camel exercise) to improve flexibility.

►Aerobic exercise (e.g., walking or swimming) to increase overall fitness and promote circulation.

Phase 3 (Chronic Phase - Functional Restoration):

► Functional strength training (e.g., squats, lunges) to target lower extremities and reduce load on the back.

► Progressive resistance training for back extensors and glutes.

► Balance and proprioception training (e.g., single-leg stance) to improve overall coordination and movement control.

4. Posture Training and Ergonomics:

Reinforced posture correction techniques during daily activities Adjustments to the workplace setup to optimize sitting posture (e.g., lumbar support, proper screen height).

5. Pain Management: Introduced modalities such as heat therapy and electrical stimulation (TENS) to reduce pain and promote relaxation.

6. Home Exercise Program:

• A customized home program focusing on core stability and lumbar flexibility.

• Daily stretching and strengthening exercises to maintain progress between sessions.

Progress Over 12 Weeks:

Weeks 1-4: Significant reduction in pain (VAS 3/10), improved posture awareness, and increased lumbar flexibility

Weeks 5-8: Gradual improvement in core strength and endurance, able to sit for longer periods without significant pain.

Weeks 9-12: Able to return to most daily activities with minimal discomfort. Functional strength improved, and patient reported better overall quality of life.

Conclusion:

Mr. J's chronic back pain was successfully managed through a combination of manual therapy, tailored exercise, ergonomic adjustments, and patient education. His pain decreased significantly, mobility and strength improved, and he regained the ability to engage in daily activities without significant limitations.

Key Takeaways:

• **Multimodal approach:** Combining manual therapy, exercise, and education was key to addressing chronic pain.

• **Patient education:** Emphasizing self-management and posture correction was crucial for long-term success

• **Tailored exercise:** A progressive exercise program addressing core weakness, flexibility, and functional movement helped restore normal function.

This case highlights the importance of a comprehensive, patient-centered approach in the physiotherapy management of chronic back pain.

: Stroke recovery with physiotherapy:

Background:

Patient Information:

Name: Mr. X

Age: 60 years

Gender: Male

Medical History: Hypertension, Type 2 Diabetes

Stroke Incident:

Type: Ischemic Stroke

Date of Stroke: February 2024 Affected Area: Right side of the brain, leading to left-sided hemiplegia (paralysis on the left side of the body)

• **Initial Symptoms:** Weakness in the left arm and leg, difficulty speaking (mild dysphasia), and facial droop on the left side.

Rehabilitation Plan:

The patient's neurologist recommended an intensive rehabilitation plan, including physiotherapy, occupational therapy, and speech therapy, with a strong emphasis on physical rehabilitation to regain motor functions.

Physiotherapy Goals:

1. **Improve Muscle Strength:** To regain movement and control over the left-sided muscles.

2. **Increase Range of Motion:** To improve the mobility of joints on the affected side.

3. **Balance and Coordination:** To prevent falls and improve independent walking.

4. **Posture and Alignment:** To correct postural imbalances due to weakness and promote proper body **mechanics.**

 5. **Gait Training:** To facilitate independent walking and reduce reliance on assistive devices.

Physiotherapy Interventions: 1. Acute Phase (1st to 2nd week post-stroke):

• **Passive Range of Motion (PROM) Exercises:** Therapists moved the

patient's limbs to maintain flexibility and prevent joint stiffness.

Positioning and Bed Mobility: Patient was taught proper positioning in bed to prevent contractures and pressure sores.

Breathing Exercises: To improve lung capacity and reduce respiratory complications.

Assisted Sitting Balance: To work on trunk control and balance while seated.

2. Sub-Acute Phase (2nd to 8th week post-stroke):

Active-Assisted Range of Motion (AAROM): The patient began participating in moving the affected limbs with assistance from the therapist.

Strengthening Exercises: Use of elastic bands and light weights to strengthen weak muscles, particularly focusing on the legs to enable walking.

 Functional Electrical Stimulation (FES): Electrical stimulation was applied to the affected muscles to improve strength and coordination.

Gait Training with Walker: The patient started walking with assistance using a walker, focusing on stepping with the left leg.

Balance Training: Exercises on a balance board and other equipment to improve standing balance and prevent falls.

 Neuromuscular Re-education: To improve the connection between the brain and the muscles, exercises were designed to stimulate motor learning and coordination.

3. Chronic Phase (3rd month onwards):

Advanced Gait Training Progressed from walker to walking with a cane, focusing on proper heel-to-toe movement.

 Proprioceptive Neuromuscular Facilitation (PNF): Techniques to improve the strength and functional use of the affected limbs.

Task-Oriented Training: The patient practiced specific tasks such as grasping objects, dressing, and climbing stairs to improve day-to-day function.

Endurance and Aerobic Exercises: To build cardiovascular fitness and overall endurance, the patient engaged in treadmill walking and stationary cycling.

Home Exercise Program: The patient was provided with a set of exercises to perform at home to maintain strength and flexibility between therapy sessions.

Outcomes:

1. Mobility: By the 6th month, the patient was able to walk independently with a cane. His gait had improved significantly, with minimal compensatory movements.

 2. Strength: The left-sided weakness had improved substantially, with 4/5 muscle strength (according to the Medical Research Council scale) in both the arm and leg.

3. Balance and Coordination: The patient regained the ability to stand independently and balance on uneven surfaces.

4. Functional Independence: The patient was able to perform activities of daily living, such as dressing, eating, and walking around the house without assistance. He continued using the cane for outdoor mobility

5. Speech and Cognition: With concurrent speech therapy, the patient's communication improved, with clear speech and the ability to participate in conversations.

Discussion:

This case highlights the importance of early and intensive physiotherapy in stroke recovery. The patient's positive outcome was attributed to a structured and goal-oriented rehabilitation plan that focused on regaining muscle strength, improving motor control, and enhancing overall functional independence. Multidisciplinary collaboration between the physiotherapist, occupational therapist, and speech therapist played a crucial role in maximizing recovery. The use of techniques like functional electrical stimulation and task-specific training was key to optimizing the rehabilitation process. Regular follow-up assessments and continued exercise programs are essential to maintain progress and prevent future complications related to stroke.

Conclusion:

Physiotherapy plays a vital role in the recovery of stroke patients, enabling them to regain mobility and independence. With consistent therapy, a tailored rehabilitation plan, and a motivated patient, significant improvements in functional outcomes. can be achieved even after a severe stroke.

D) Case study 3: Post-operative rehabilitation for joint replacement :-

Patient Background:

• **Name:** Mr. D

• **Age:** 65 years

• **Medical History:** Osteoarthritis of the right knee, controlled hypertension, mild obesity (BMI 29), and a history of smoking (quit 5 years ago).

• **Surgical Procedure:** Total Knee Replacement (TKR) on the right knee due to progressive osteoarthritis, significantly affecting mobility and quality of life.

• **Preoperative Condition:** Mr. D presented with severe pain in the right knee, decreased range of motion, and significant difficulties in walking or standing for prolonged periods. Conservative treatments like medication, physical therapy, and injections provided only temporary relief.

Post-Operative Rehabilitation Plan:

1. Immediate Post-Op Care (Day 1-3):

• **Pain Management:** The patient received opioid analgesics for pain control and was closely monitored for any side effects. A continuous passive motion (CPM) machine was used to reduce stiffness.

• **Early Mobilization:** On post-op day 1, the patient was encouraged to sit up and stand with assistance using a walker. Physical therapy started with gentle range of motion (ROM) exercises to prevent stiffness and blood clots.

• **Deep Breathing Exercises:** To prevent post-operative pneumonia, the patient practiced breathing exercises with a spirometer.

2. Week 1-2: Early Rehabilitation:-

Physical Therapy: Twice daily sessions focused on increasing range of motion, regaining strength, and promoting early weight-bearing (as tolerated). Exercises included: Ankle pumps to improve circulation.

• Quad sets (isometric quadriceps contractions).

• Assisted leg lifts and gentle bending of the knee.

• Heel slides to promote flexion and extension.

Cryotherapy: Ice was applied to the knee for swelling and pain management after exercises.

Wound Care: Monitoring for signs of infection and ensuring proper healing.

3. Week 3-6: Intermediate Rehabilitation

• **Strengthening and Mobility:** The patient progressed to more advanced exercises such as:

- Stationary biking (low resistance).

- Partial squats and step-ups to improve strength.

- Use of resistance bands for quadriceps and hamstring strengthening.

Gait Training: Focused on improving walking mechanics and reducing the reliance on assistive devices (e.g... cane or walker).

Balance Training: Introducing balance exercises to prevent falls and improve proprioception.

Pain Control: Transitioning to non-opioid medications (NSAIDs) as pain subsided.

4. Week 7-12: Advanced Rehabilitation

- **Full-Weight Bearing:** Patient was encouraged to walk independently, with minimal assistance from a cane. Full weight-bearing on the operated leg was achieved.

- **Range of Motion:** The goal was to reach 120 degrees of knee flexion. Stretching exercises were introduced.

- **Strengthening and Endurance:** More complex exercises such as lunges, cycling, and swimming were integrated. Resistance increased for leg presses and step exercises.

- **Return to Activities:** Low-impact activities like swimming or walking were recommended to maintain fitness without stressing the joint.

5. Long-Term Rehabilitation (3-12 months):

- **Functional Training:** Focused on returning to daily activities, such as climbing stairs, driving, and recreational activities.

- **Monitoring for Complications:** Regular follow-ups to ensure there were no signs of infection, prosthesis issues, or deep vein thrombosis. (DVT).

Outcomes:

By 6 months post-op, John achieved near full range of motion, with 120 degrees of knee flexion and extension.

- He was able to walk independently without pain, return to recreational activities, and perform daily tasks without difficulty. Strengthening and endurance exercises were continued as part of a maintenance plan.

on individual goals and limitations.

This case highlights the importance of a multi-disciplinary approach, involving surgeons, physical therapists, and nursing staff to optimize post-operative recovery.

E) Case study 4: Sports injury recovery using physiotherapy :-

Introduction: Sports injuries are common across all levels of physical activity, ranging from minor sprains to serious conditions like ligament tears or fractures, Physiotherapy plays a pivotal role in the rehabilitation and recovery of athletes by helping restore movement, strength, and functionality while preventing future injuries.

Patient Profile:

- **Name: Mr. R**

- **Age: 28**

- **Sport: Football (Amateur Level) Injury:** ACL (Anterior Cruciate Ligament) Tear

- **Background:** Mr.R sustained an ACL tear during a football match after an awkward landing following a jump.

This injury typically requires surgical intervention, followed by an extensive rehabilitation program to regain full knee function.

Initial Assessment:

Pain Level: 8/10 (in the acute phase) Swelling: Significant around the knee joint

Range of Motion: Severely restricted. unable to fully extend or bend the knee

Strength: Weakness in the quadriceps and hamstring muscles, which support the knee joint

Physiotherapy Objectives:

1. Reduce pain and swelling.

2. Restore full range of motion in the knee.

3. Strengthen muscles surrounding the knee

4. Improve balance and coordination to prevent future injuries.

5. Return to sport safely and gradually.

Phase 1: Acute Phase (0-2 Weeks Post-Surgery)

Goals:

- Minimize swelling and pain.

- Begin gentle mobility exercises.

Intervention:

Cryotherapy: Ice packs were applied several times a day to control swelling and pain.

Compression and Elevation: Use of a compression bandage and keeping the leg elevated to manage swelling.

Manual Therapy: Gentle massage around the knee to improve circulation and reduce stiffness.

Passive Range of Motion (PROM): With assistance, the knee was moved within a pain-free range to prevent stiffness and improve mobility.

Outcome: By the end of the second week, the swelling reduced, and John was able to bend his knee to 90 degrees.

Phase 2: Sub-Acute Phase (2-6 Weeks Post-Surgery)

Goals:

• Increase range of motion

• Start strengthening exercises without stressing the ligament repair.

Intervention:

Active Range of Motion (AROM): Mr. R started to perform knee flexion and extension exercises under supervision to gradually increase his range of motion.

• **Quadriceps and Hamstring Activation:** Isometric exercises (contracting muscles without moving the joint) were introduced to start building muscle strength without putting stress on the knee.

• **Cycling:** Low-resistance stationary cycling to enhance knee mobility and blood flow to the area.

Outcome: At the end of six weeks, Mr. R regained about 80% of his knee's range of motion and showed signs of muscle strength returning.

Phase 3: Strengthening and Proprioception (6-12 Weeks Post-Surgery)

Goals:

• Build strength in the quadriceps, hamstrings, and calf muscles.

• Improve balance and proprioception.

Intervention:

• **Strength Training:** Exercises such as leg presses, squats, and hamstring curls were added with light weights to progressively build strength in the knee and supporting muscles.

• **Balance Training:** Mr. R was introduced to single-leg stands, balance boards, and foam pads to improve his coordination and proprioception (the body's ability to sense movement and position).

• **Core Stability:** Core exercises were also integrated to enhance overall body stability, which helps in preventing future injuries.

• **Outcome:** By the 12th week, Mr. R demonstrated a marked improvement in muscle strength and balance, with nearly full range of motion restored.

Phase 4: Return to Sport-Specific Training (12-20 Weeks Post-Surgery)

Goals:

• Prepare for return to sports by mimicking football-specific movements.

• Ensure full recovery of knee function under dynamic conditions.

Intervention:

• **Agility Drills:** Ladder drills, side shuffles, and forward-backward running exercises were incorporated to mimic the movements required in football.

• **Plyometric Training :**

Low-intensity jumping and landing exercises were added to prepare John's knee for the stresses of sports activities.

• **Gradual Sport Resumption:**

Controlled practice sessions were introduced with limited playtime and no contact, allowing the knee to adapt to sports-specific demands.

• **Outcome:** By the end of this phase, Mr. R returned to light football training with no pain, full range of motion, and sufficient strength.

Phase 5: Full Return to Sport (20+ Weeks Post-Surgery)

Goals:

• Safely reintegrate into full-contact football.

• Maintain strength and flexibility to prevent reinjury.

Intervention:

Full Sports Drills: Mr. R participated in full-contact football training and practice sessions with ongoing monitoring from his physiotherapist.

 Maintenance Program: A long-term strengthening and flexibility program was provided to ensure his knee remained strong and injury-free, including strength training, balance issues.

Conclusion: Physiotherapy was integral to Mr. R's recovery from an ACL tear, aiding in his return to sport while minimizing the risk of future injury. The structured, phased approach ensured that each aspect of his recovery, from pain management to sport-specific training, was addressed comprehensively. A combination of manual therapy, strengthening, mobility work, and proprioception training allowed Mr. R to regain full function and return to his pre-injury performance level in football.

F) Case study 5: Pediatric physiotherapy success story :-

Name: Sarah

Age: 4 years old

Condition: Cerebral Palsy (Spastic Diplegia)

Sarah was diagnosed with spastic diplegia, a form of cerebral palsy, at the age of 18 months. This condition primarily affected her lower limbs, leading to stiff muscles and difficulty walking. Her family sought physiotherapy intervention to help her improve mobility and gain independence.

Initial Assessment:

During Sarah's first physiotherapy assessment, she presented with:

Limited mobility: Unable to stand or walk independently.

Muscle stiffness: Especially in her hips, knees, and ankles.

Delayed motor skills: Difficulty with balance, coordination, and fine motor tasks.

Emotional frustration: Due to limited ability to interact with peers.

A team consisting of a pediatric physiotherapist, occupational therapist, and a speech therapist created an individualized treatment plan.

Treatment Plan

The goal was to improve Sarah's motor functions, strengthen muscles, and help her achieve basic mobility. The treatment plan was tailored for her developmental stage and involved the following components:

1. Stretching and Strengthening Exercises

Daily exercises targeting her lower limbs to reduce stiffness and improve muscle strength, especially focusing on hip abductors, hamstrings, and calf muscles.

2. Gait Training

The therapist used a combination of parallel bars, gait trainers, and later, lightweight orthotics to assist Sarah in standing and walking. Sessions focused on improving her weight-bearing ability and teaching her how to shift her balance for better movement,

3. Hydrotherapy

Water-based exercises were introduced to make movement easier and more enjoyable for Sarah. The buoyancy of water helped reduce the impact of gravity on her limbs, allowing her to practice walking movements in a low-resistance environment.

4. Play Therapy

To engage Sarah in therapy, play-based approaches were used. Games involving ball-throwing, jumping, and crawling helped her improve coordination while keeping her motivated and enthusiastic about therapy.

5. Parental Involvement

Sarah's parents were educated on the importance of continuing therapy at home. The physiotherapist provided a series of at-home exercises, along with guidance on how to encourage Sarah during everyday activities to further promote independence.

Progress and Outcomes

After 12 months of consistent therapy, Sarah showed remarkable improvement:

• **Increased Mobility:** Sarah could now stand independently and take 10-15 steps without support. With a walker, she could cover longer distances.

• **Improved Muscle Tone:** Regular stretching helped reduce stiffness in her lower limbs, and her range of motion increased significantly.

• **Enhanced Motor Skills:** Sarah's coordination and balance improved, allowing her to participate in more play activities with her peers.

• **Emotional Growth:** The improvement in her physical abilities had a positive effect on her emotional well-being. She became more confident and socially engaged with children her age.

Conclusion

Sarah's success story highlights the importance of early intervention in pediatric physiotherapy. Through a combination of stretching, strengthening, gait training, and family involvement, Sarah was able to achieve milestones that greatly improved her quality of life. While she will likely continue therapy as she grows, her progress has set a strong foundation for future development.

This case demonstrates how personalized physiotherapy treatment can make a significant difference in the lives of children with physical disabilities.

10. Future of Physiotherapy:-

A)Advancements in technology (telehealth, wearable devices) :-

The future of physiotherapy is poised for significant advancements driven by technology, promising more personalized, efficient, and accessible treatment options. Here are some key areas of technological progress:

1. Wearable Devices and Sensors

• **Real-time Monitoring:** Wearable devices equipped with sensors can monitor a patient's movement, posture, and physical activity in real time. These devices provide continuous feedback, allowing physiotherapists to make more informed treatment decisions.

• **Injury Prevention:** Data from wearables can predict the likelihood of injury by tracking movement patterns, helping in early intervention and reducing the risk of injury recurrence.

2. Tele-rehabilitation

• **Remote Consultations:** Telehealth technologies are enabling patients to receive physiotherapy remotely. This is particularly useful for individuals in rural or underserved areas, and also for those with mobility challenges.

Virtual Home Exercises: Through video conferencing and specialized apps, physiotherapists can guide patients through their exercises remotely while ensuring they perform them correctly.

3. Artificial Intelligence (AI) and Machine Learning

• **Data-Driven Insights:** AI can analyze data from patient histories, wearable devices, and imaging to offer predictive insights, helping physiotherapists to customize treatment plans.

• **Virtual Assistants:** AI-based virtual assistants can help guide patients through rehabilitation exercises, ensuring proper technique and form, potentially reducing the need for frequent in-person visits.

4. Robotics and Exoskeletons

Rehabilitation Robotics:

Robots designed for physical therapy are becoming more common in aiding movement and muscle retraining, especially for patients recovering from strokes or serious injuries.

- **Exoskeletons:** Wearable robotic exoskeletons help patients with paralysis or severe mobility issues regain some movement. These devices can aid in gait training and other forms of physical therapy, offering hope to those with spinal cord injuries or neurological conditions.

5. Virtual Reality (VR) and Augmented Reality (AR)

- **Immersive Therapy:** VR is being used to create immersive environments that can help patients regain motor skills through simulated exercises. These virtual environments provide motivation and engagement while facilitating recovery.

- **AR for Guidance:** AR can overlay real-time information on a patient's body during exercises, guiding them to correct movements and postures during rehabilitation.

6. 3D Printing

Custom Orthotics and Prosthetics: 3D printing allows for the creation of highly customized prosthetics and orthotic devices that are perfectly. tailored to the patient's anatomy. These devices enhance the comfort and effectiveness of physiotherapy for those with limb impairments.

 Assistive Devices: The ability to quickly prototype assistive devices for patients also allows for faster and more cost-effective solutions.

7. Advanced Imaging and Biomechanics

- **Movement Analysis:** Advanced motion capture and imaging technologies can assess a patient's biomechanics in detail, identifying subtle imbalances or weaknesses. This data helps create more targeted treatment plans.

- **Ultrasound and MRI:** Improved imaging technologies allow physiotherapists to visualize soft tissue injuries more clearly, which can guide more precise and effective interventions.

8.Personalized Treatment Plans

- **Genomics and Precision Medicine:** Emerging fields like genomics may eventually allow for more personalized physiotherapy approaches based on a patient's genetic predisposition to certain Injuries or recovery pathways.

- **Customized Exercise Plans:** Machine learning algorithms can analyze patient data to design exercise regimens that are specifically optimized for the individual's recovery needs and physical condition.

9. Automation and AI-assisted Documentation

Efficiency in Practice: AI tools can assist in automating patient documentation and administrative. tasks, freeing up more time for physiotherapists to focus on patient care.

Data-Driven Adjustments: AI can help track patient progress and adjust treatment plans based on real-time data, improving outcomes.

10. Gamification

- **Motivational Tools:** Gamifying physiotherapy exercises can improve patient compliance. Through the integration of video game elements, patients are more engaged in their rehabilitation process, which often leads to faster recovery times.

These advancements in technology are not only improving treatment outcomes but also making physiotherapy more accessible and efficient. The future of physiotherapy will likely see a continued blending of human expertise with cutting-edge technology, enhancing the quality of patient care.

B) Integration of AI in physiotherapy treatments :-

Integrating AI into physiotherapy treatments involves combining advanced technology with traditional physical therapy to enhance diagnosis, treatment planning, and patient outcomes. Here are some key ways AI is being integrated into physiotherapy:

1.Assessment and Diagnosis:

• AI can analyze patient data, such as movement patterns and posture, using wearable sensors and cameras. These devices can provide detailed insights into the range of motion, joint angles, and muscle activation, helping physiotherapists make more accurate diagnoses.

• Machine learning algorithms can predict injury risks by analyzing biomechanical data, improving early intervention and treatment.

2. Personalized Treatment Plans:

• AI algorithms can tailor physiotherapy programs based on patient-specific data, including medical history, current physical abilities, and progress. These programs can adapt dynamically as the patient improves, ensuring that the treatment is both effective and efficient.

• Virtual AI assistants can guide patients through exercises, offering real-time feedback on their form and technique to ensure they are performing movements correctly.

3. Remote Monitoring and Tele-rehabilitation:

• AI-driven apps and platforms allow patients to receive remote physiotherapy. Using motion-tracking technology and machine learning, these platforms can monitor patients' exercises at home, providing instant feedback and corrections.

• AI can track a patient's progress and suggest adjustments to their therapy regimen based on data collected over time, enabling continuous care outside of clinical settings.

4. Rehabilitation Robotics:

• AI-powered exoskeletons and rehabilitation robots can assist patients with limited mobility. These devices use AI to adapt to the patient's movements and needs, providing support and resistance as required, which accelerates recovery.

5. Predictive Analytics:

• AI can predict the likelihood of patient recovery timelines and outcomes, based on data patterns from previous patients. This can help physiotherapists manage patient expectations and adjust treatment plans accordingly.

6. Gamification of Therapy:

• AI-driven platforms can incorporate gamification into physiotherapy exercises, making the rehabilitation process more engaging for patients, especially for children or those undergoing long-term therapy.

7. Virtual Reality (VR) and Augmented Reality (AR):

• AI is integrated with VR/AR systems to create immersive rehabilitation environments, speech rehabilitation is required, AI-driven tools can analyze speech patterns, facial movements, and cognitive responses to offer targeted exercises and track improvements over time.

The integration of AI in physiotherapy is set to transform rehabilitation by making it more personalized, accessible, and data-driven, improving both the patient experience and therapeutic outcomes.

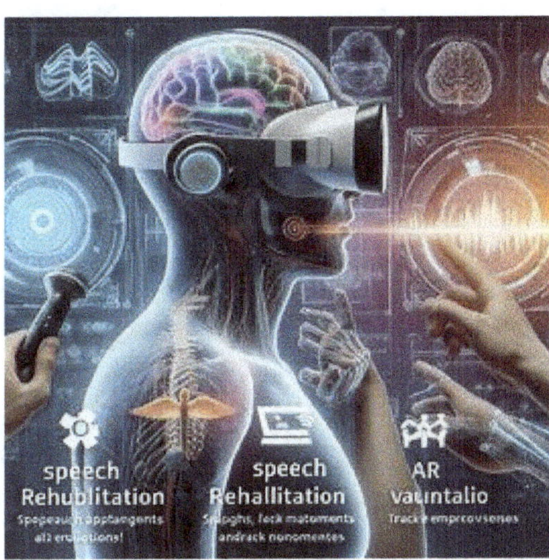

C) Innovations in rehabilitation techniques:-

Innovation in rehabilitation techniques is transforming how patients recover from injuries, surgeries, and chronic conditions. Recent advancements include the integration of technology, data-driven approaches, and personalized therapies, making rehabilitation more efficient and accessible. Key innovations include:

1. Robotics and Exoskeletons:

• Robotic devices assist in movement therapy, helping individuals with physical impairments regain mobility. Exoskeletons can enable patients to walk again, even after severe spinal injuries or strokes.

• Upper-limb rehabilitation robots aid patients recovering from arm injuries or neurological conditions, offering tailored and repetitive movements to regain strength and control.

2. Virtual Reality (VR) and Augmented Reality (AR):

• VR and AR create immersive environments where patients can perform exercises that are more engaging and enjoyable. This increases motivation and enhances motor skill recovery, especially in stroke and neurological rehabilitation.

• **Gamification** of physical therapy is another growing trend, where patients interact with virtual environments to perform prescribed exercises, which can improve adherence to rehabilitation plans.

3. Telerehabilitation:

• With the rise of telehealth, telerehabilitation allows patients to perform therapy at home under remote supervision from clinicians. This approach is especially beneficial in rural or underserved areas where access to rehabilitation centers is limited.

- Wearable devices, mobile apps, and motion sensors can track a patient's progress in real time, allowing therapists to adjust treatment protocols accordingly.

4. 3D Printing and Custom Orthotics:

- 3D printing is being used to create personalized prosthetics and orthotic. devices that perfectly match a patient's anatomy, improving comfort and functionality.

- These innovations allow for faster production of custom aids, from splints to braces, which can be tailored for specific rehabilitation needs.

5. Neuroplasticity-Based Therapies:

- New treatments focus on harnessing the brain's ability to rewire itself, known as neuroplasticity. Techniques like constraint-induced movement therapy (CIMT) force the use of an impaired limb to encourage recovery in stroke patients.

- Non-invasive brain stimulation, such as transcranial magnetic stimulation. (TMS), is also being explored to improve motor recovery and cognitive function.

6. Artificial Intelligence and Machine Learning:

- AI is increasingly used to analyze patient data, predict recovery patterns, and customize rehabilitation. protocols. Machine learning models. can predict which interventions will be most effective for specific injuries or conditions, optimizing care pathways.

- Rehabilitation robots powered by AI can adjust to a patient's progress,

delivering more personalized and effective therapy.

7. Biofeedback and Wearable Technology:

- Wearable sensors and biofeedback devices provide real-time data on a patient's movements, muscle activity, and posture. This technology helps patients adjust their form and performance during exercises.

- **Smart garments** embedded with sensors track rehabilitation progress and can send feedback to therapists, enhancing personalized therapy at home.

8. Hydrotherapy and Aquatic Therapy Innovations:

- Innovations in water-based therapy. include advanced underwater treadmills and water-resistant resistance bands. These tools leverage the buoyancy and resistance of water to help patients rehabilitate without putting excessive strain on their joints.

9. Stem Cell Therapy and Regenerative Medicine:

Stem cells and regenerative techniques are being explored to treat muscle, cartilage, and nerve damage. While still in experimental stages,

- FES uses electrical impulses to stimulate muscles, helping individuals with paralysis or significant weakness regain movement. This technique is commonly used for spinal cord injury patients and in post-stroke rehabilitation to enhance motor recovery.

These innovations are not only improving patient outcomes but also making rehabilitation more engaging, efficient, and accessible. The future of rehabilitation will likely see even greater integration of technology and personalized care approaches.

D) Global trends in physiotherapy education and practice :-

Global trends in physiotherapy education and practice are evolving rapidly, shaped by advancements in healthcare, technology, and shifting patient demographics. Here are key trends influencing the field:

1. Expansion of Entry-Level Doctoral Programs

Many countries, especially in North America, are transitioning to Doctor of Physical Therapy (DPT) as the entry-level qualification. This reflects the increasing complexity of clinical knowledge required for physiotherapists and the growing demand for higher education standards.

2. Evidence-Based Practice

• The emphasis on evidence-based practice (EBP) is driving physiotherapy education globally. Institutions are increasingly. integrating research methods, critical appraisal, and clinical reasoning into curricula, encouraging students to base their clinical decisions on solid scientific evidence.

• Practitioners are expected to continually update their knowledge based on current research to improve patient outcomes.

3. Use of Technology and Telehealth

Telehealth and virtual physiotherapy have grown significantly, especially post-COVID-19, allowing for remote patient consultations, assessments, and treatment plans. Wearable technology, apps for remote monitoring, and gamified rehabilitation tools are becoming part of standard practice, promoting patient engagement and tracking real-time progress.

4. Interdisciplinary and Collaborative Care

• The role of physiotherapists within multidisciplinary teams is expanding. They are increasingly working. alongside other healthcare professionals (e.g., doctors, occupational therapists, and psychologists) to offer more holistic care.

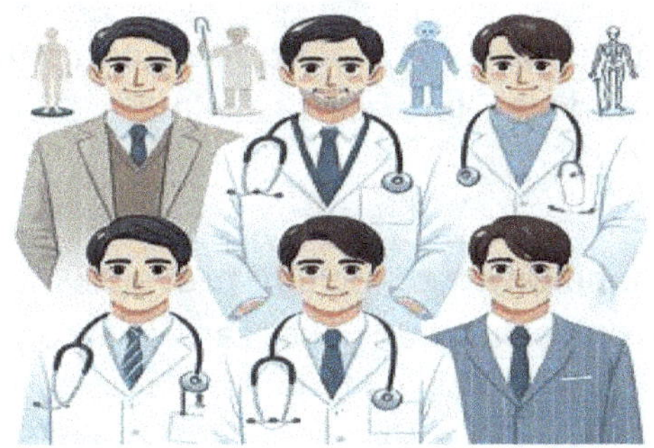

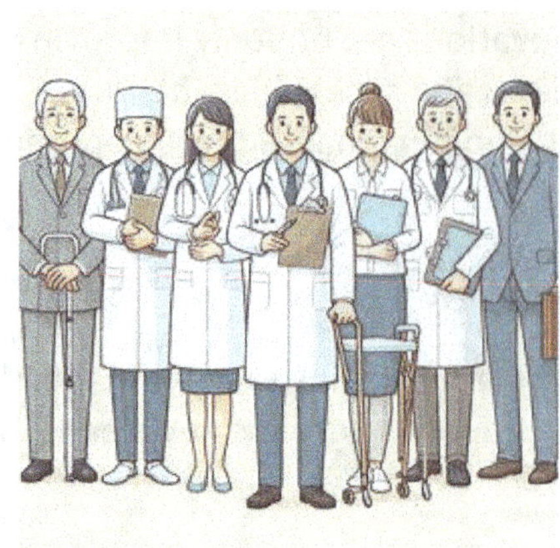

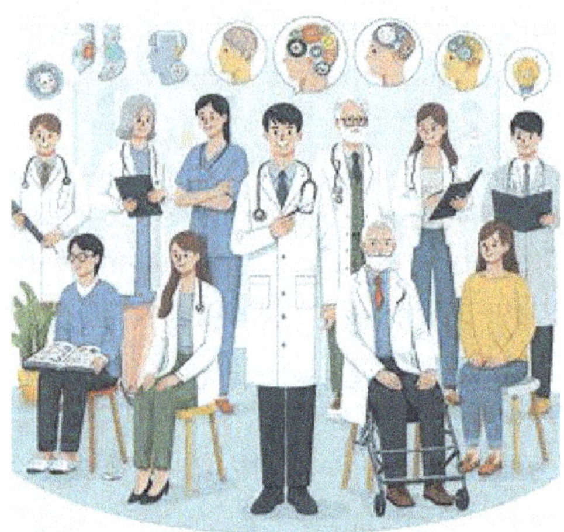

• This is particularly evident in fields. like sports medicine, neurology, and geriatrics, where complex cases benefit from a team-based approach.

5. Global Standardization of Education

• Organizations like the World Confederation for Physical Therapy (WCPT) advocate for the global standardization of physiotherapy education to ensure high-quality care worldwide. Countries are gradually aligning their curricula to meet these international benchmarks.

• This movement also promotes cross-border opportunities for practitioners and students, with increased emphasis on global exchange programs and standardized licensing.

6. Focus on Preventive Care and Wellness

• Physiotherapy is increasingly moving beyond rehabilitation to include preventive care, focusing on overall wellness, fitness, and the prevention of chronic conditions like. cardiovascular diseases, diabetes, and musculoskeletal issues.

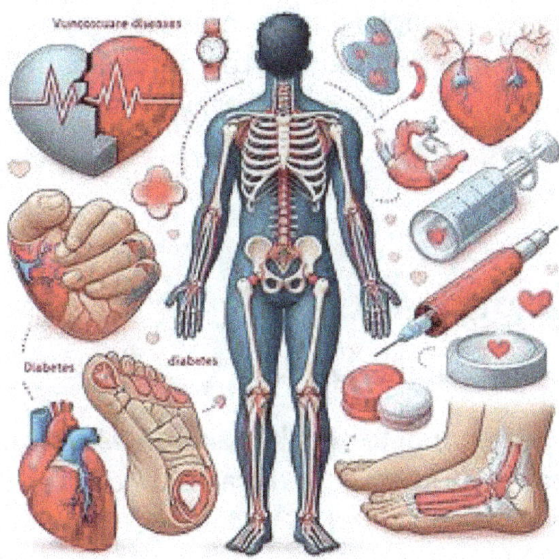

• Education programs are incorporating more public health components, training physiotherapists to work in settings like schools, workplaces, and communities to prevent injury and promote health.

7. Manual Therapy vs. Technology Integration

• While manual therapy remains a cornerstone of physiotherapy practice, there is an ongoing debate about balancing traditional techniques with modern technology.

• In some regions, there's a push toward high-tech approaches like robotic rehabilitation, virtual reality (VR) for pain management, and artificial intelligence (AI) for diagnostic support.

8. Cultural Competence and Diversity in Practice

• As healthcare becomes more globalized, there is a growing. emphasis on training physiotherapists in cultural competence. This ensures they can effectively serve diverse **populations with different health beliefs and practices.**

• Programs are increasingly including modules on addressing health disparities, understanding global health systems, and providing culturally sensitive care.

9. Specialization and Advanced Practice Roles

• There is a rise in specialization within physiotherapy, with professionals seeking advanced certifications in areas like orthopedic manual therapy, sports physiotherapy, neurorehabilitation, and pediatric care.

• Some countries are also recognizing advanced practice physiotherapists (APPs), who can perform expanded roles such as prescribing medications, ordering diagnostic tests, or performing certain interventions.

10. Sustainability and Green Healthcare Initiatives

• The trend towards environmentally sustainable healthcare practices is also impacting physiotherapy. Clinics and educational institutions are adopting sustainable practices, such as reducing waste, using eco-friendly equipment, and promoting sustainable travel for home-based therapy.

These trends highlight the increasing complexity, scope, and professionalism in physiotherapy education and practice, helping to improve patient outcomes and broaden the reach of physiotherapy across healthcare systems globally.

11. How to Choose the Right Physiotherapist:-

A) Qualifications and certifications to look for physiotherapy :-

 When seeking a qualified physiotherapist, it's essential to check their educational background, certifications, and licensing. Here are key qualifications and certificates to look for:

1. Educational Qualifications

Bachelor's Degree in Physiotherapy (BPT): This is a minimum requirement for becoming a licensed physiotherapist in many countries. The degree typically takes 4-5 years.

Master's Degree in Physiotherapy (MPT in Physiotherapy): A postgraduate degree specializing in fields like orthopedics, sports, neurology, pediatrics, or cardiovascular physiotherapy can indicate advanced knowledge.

2. Certifications

State/Regional License: Ensure the physiotherapist is licensed to practice in your area. This usually involves passing an exam after completing their degree.

Specialty Certifications: Depending on their area of focus, physiotherapists may hold additional certifications, such as:

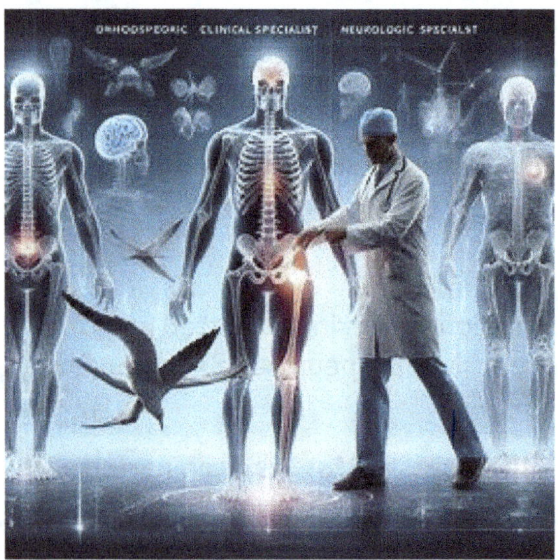

- Orthopedic Clinical Specialist (OCS)

- Neurologic Clinical Specialist (NCS)

- Sports Physiotherapy Certification

- Manual Therapy Certifications: Techniques like Maitland, McKenzie, or Mulligan.

- Dry Needling Certification: If they offer dry needling as part of their treatment.

3. Continuing Education & Memberships

Continuing Professional Development (CPD): Many physiotherapists are required to regularly update their skills through workshops, courses, or seminars.

Professional Memberships: Beingpart of a recognized physiotherapy association.

Always verify their credentials with the appropriate licensing body to ensure they are in good standing.

B) Questions to ask during the consultation :-

When visiting a physiotherapist, asking the right questions ensures that you understand your condition and the treatment plan. Here are some useful questions to ask:

1. Understanding Your Condition:

• What is the cause of my pain or injury?

• Can you explain my diagnosis in simple terms?

• How long will it take to recover?

2. Treatment Plan:

• What treatment options are available for my condition?

• How often do I need to come for therapy sessions?

• What will the therapy sessions involve?

• Will I need any special equipment for exercises at home?

3. Expected Outcomes:

• What results can I expect from this treatment?

• Are there any alternative treatments or therapies I should consider?

• How can I monitor my progress?

4. Pain and Activity Management:

• Should I avoid certain activities or movements during treatment?

• What can I do to manage pain at home?

• Are there any stretches or exercises I should do regularly?

5. Long-term Care and Prevention:

or body mechanics to avoid future issues?

6. Medical Referrals and Further Testing:

• Do I need a referral to a specialist or any further testing (e.g., MRI, X-ray)?

• Should I consider seeing a chiropractor, osteopath, or other healthcare providers?

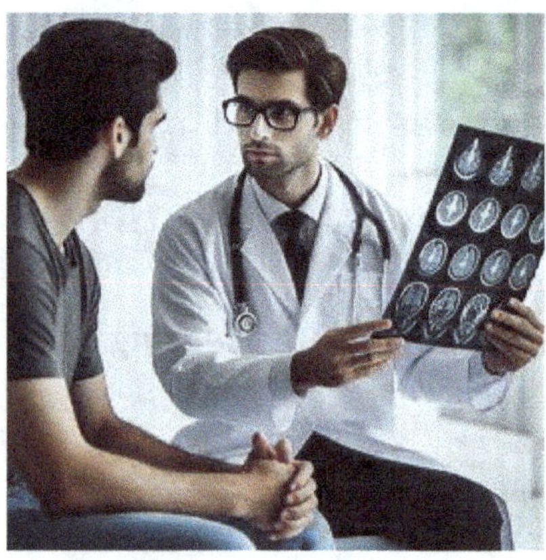

Asking these questions will help you have a clearer understanding of your therapy and recovery process.

C) Red flags to avoid :-

When choosing a physiotherapist or undergoing physiotherapy treatment, it's important to watch out for certain red flags that may indicate poor practice or risk of harm.

1. Lack of Proper Qualifications :-

Ensure the physiotherapist is licensed and registered with a recognized physiotherapy board or regulatory body. Unqualified or uncertified practitioners may lack the skills and knowledge necessary for safe treatment.

2. No Initial Assessment or Diagnosis :-

• A good physiotherapist will start with a thorough assessment of your condition, medical history, and physical limitations. If they skip this step and jump straight into treatment, it's a sign of unprofessional practice.

3. One-Size-Fits-All Approach :-

Physiotherapy should be personalized to your specific needs. Be cautious if the therapist uses the same exercises or treatment plans for everyone without considering your unique condition.

4. Pain During Treatment :-

While some discomfort can be normal. during physiotherapy, especially in the case of stretching or deep tissue massage, persistent pain during or after treatment is a red flag. Your therapist should adjust the treatment if it's causing significant pain.

5. Overuse of Passive Treatments :-

• Be wary if the therapist heavily relies on passive treatments (e.g., ultrasound, heat therapy, electrical stimulation) without incorporating active rehabilitation exercises or manual therapy. Passive treatments. should supplement, not replace, active recovery.

6. No Progress Tracking or Adjustments :-

• If your treatment plan doesn't evolve or the therapist doesn't track your progress over time, it suggests poor quality of care. Therapy should be dynamic, with regular reassessments and adjustments to the plan based on your progress.

7. Pushing for Expensive or Excessive Sessions :-

• Some therapists may push for too many sessions or treatments you don't need. Be cautious if they seem more interested in selling packages or expensive treatments rather than focusing on your recovery goals.

8. Poor Communication or Dismissiveness :-

• A physiotherapist who doesn't listen to your concerns or dismisses your pain and experiences may not be offering appropriate care. Good communication and understanding are key to effective treatment.

9. Unclear or Unproven Techniques :-

• If the physiotherapist uses unconventional or experimental treatments without evidence-based pose health risks.

By being aware of these red flags, you can better ensure you receive high-quality, safe physiotherapy care.

D) Understanding the treatment plan and setting realistic goals :-

Understanding a treatment plan and setting realistic goals in physiotherapy is essential for maximizing recovery and maintaining motivation.

1. Assessment and Diagnosis :-

The first step in physiotherapy involves a detailed assessment of your condition. The physiotherapist evaluates your physical limitations, pain, strength, flexibility, and mobility. Based on this, they create a diagnosis and identify the root cause of your issues, whether it's related to muscles, joints, nerves, or other systems.

2. Understanding the Treatment Plan :-

Individualized Approach:

Physiotherapy treatment plans are tailored to the individual, considering the specific condition, goals, lifestyle, and physical capacity.

Therapy Modalities: Common treatments may include manual therapy, exercises, stretches, electrotherapy, or heat/cold therapy. The purpose of each modality should be explained to you, so you understand how it contributes to your recovery.

Frequency and Duration: The plan outlines how many sessions you need per week and how long the overall treatment is expected to last. The physiotherapist may adjust this based on your progress.

3. Setting Realistic Goals :-

Short-term vs. Long-term Goals: Short-term goals are smaller milestones (e.g., reducing pain, regaining a specific range of motion), while long-term goals aim at full recovery (e.g., returning to sports or normal activities).

SMART Goals: Goals in physiotherapy are often set using the SMART criteria -Specific, Measurable, Achievable, Relevant, and Time-bound. For example, "Increase knee flexion by 20 degrees within 4 weeks."

Collaboration: Discuss goals with your physiotherapist to ensure they align with your expectations and lifestyle. Goals should be challenging but attainable, factoring in the severity of your condition and the body's natural healing process.

4. Adherence and Self-management

Home Exercise Program: Most physiotherapy plans include exercises to do at home. Adhering to these routines is crucial for faster recovery.

Feedback Loop: Regularly communicate with your physiotherapist about how your body feels, any progress, or new challenges. They can modify the treatment if necessary.

5. Tracking Progress

Measurements: Physiotherapists track progress using objective measures such as range of motion, strength tests, pain scales, and functional tests.

Celebrating Milestones: Acknowledge small improvements to stay motivated. Even incremental progress, like being able to walk without pain or lift a heavier weight, is a step forward.

fluctuations in pain or progress.

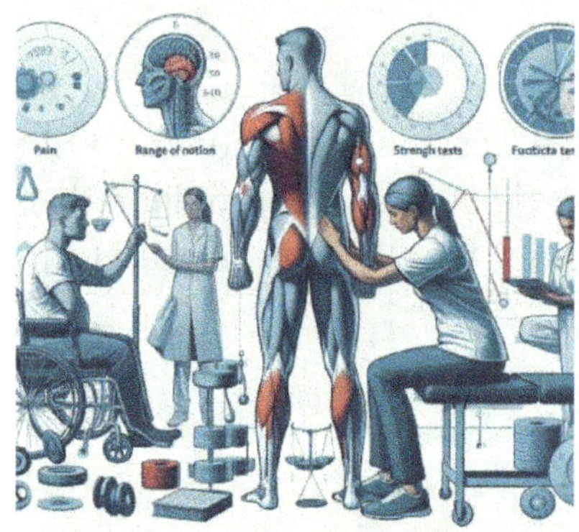

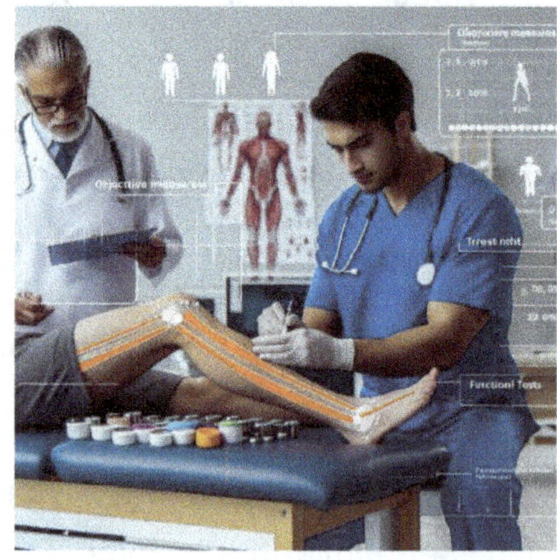

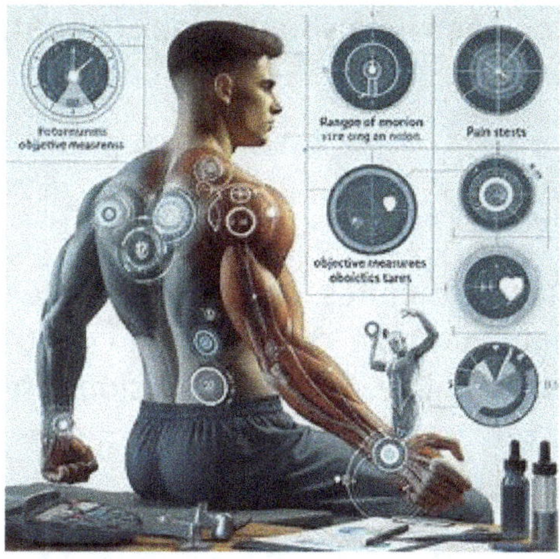

Conclusion :-

Understanding your treatment plan and setting realistic goals in physiotherapy requires a balance of professional guidance and self-commitment. Being proactive, maintaining clear communication, and setting achievable goals with your physiotherapist will help optimize your recovery process.

12. Frequently Asked Questions (FAQ) About Physiotherapy:-

A)What can I expect during my first physiotherapy session?

During your first physiotherapy session, you can expect the following:

1. Initial Assessment: The physiotherapist will ask about your medical history, symptoms, pain levels, and the goals you hope to achieve with physiotherapy. They may inquire about daily activities, previous injuries, or conditions affecting your mobility.

2. Physical Examination: The physiotherapist will assess your posture, range of motion, strength, flexibility, and balance. They may ask you to perform specific movements to observe how your body responds.

3. Diagnosis and Plan: Based on the assessment, the physiotherapist will explain their diagnosis and develop a tailored treatment plan. This plan may include exercises, stretches, or other therapies to help you recover or improve your condition.

4. Demonstration of Exercises: You'll likely be shown some basic exercises or stretches to start with, which you can also do at home. These exercises will target areas that need strengthening, flexibility, or pain relief.

6. Education and Advice: The physiotherapist may give advice on posture, ergonomics, or lifestyle adjustments to help manage your condition or prevent further injury.

7. Duration and Follow-up: Your session could last between 30-60 minutes, and the therapist will likely schedule follow-up sessions depending on the severity of your condition and the treatment plan.

It's important to wear comfortable clothing and be open with your therapist about any discomfort during the session.

B) How long do physiotherapy sessions typically last?

Physiotherapy sessions typically last between 30 to 60 minutes, depending on the type of therapy and the patient's specific needs. Initial assessments may take longer, around 45 to 90 minutes, as the therapist needs time to evaluate your condition thoroughly. Follow-up sessions are often shorter but can vary based on the treatment plan.

C) How many sessions do I need?

The number of sessions you need in physiotherapy depends on several factors, including:

1. Nature of the Injury or Condition: Minor issues may only require a few sessions, while more severe injuries or chronic conditions could take several weeks or months.

2. Your Personal Goals: Some people may continue physiotherapy after their injury heals to maintain strength or prevent future problems.

3. Body's Response to Treatment: Healing rates vary from person to person, and your physiotherapist will assess how your body responds over time.

4. Type of Treatment: Some treatments, like post-surgery recovery, may require more frequent and longer-term sessions.

It's best to follow your physiotherapist's recommendations, as they will create a personalized treatment plan based on your specific needs. A common approach might involve 6-12 sessions for moderate conditions, but it could be shorter or longer depending on progress.

D) Is physiotherapy painful?

Physiotherapy is not typically painful, though it can sometimes cause discomfort, especially when working with injured or stiff areas. The goal of physiotherapy is to improve movement, strength, and function while managing pain, not increasing it. However, some people may experience mild soreness or discomfort during or after certain exercises or treatments, similar to the sensation of having exercised after a long break.

Your physiotherapist should tailor the intensity of treatment to your pain tolerance, and it's important to communicate with them if you're feeling too much pain so adjustments can be made.

E) Can physiotherapy help with chronic conditions?

Yes, physiotherapy can be very helpful in managing chronic conditions. It can improve mobility, reduce pain, enhance strength, and restore function over time. Physiotherapists use tailored exercise programs, manual therapy, and various techniques like electrotherapy or heat/ cold therapy to treat chronic conditions. Some common chronic conditions where physiotherapy is effective include:

1. Arthritis - Reduces joint pain, improves flexibility, and enhances mobility.

2. Chronic back pain - Helps to strengthen muscles, improve posture, and manage pain.

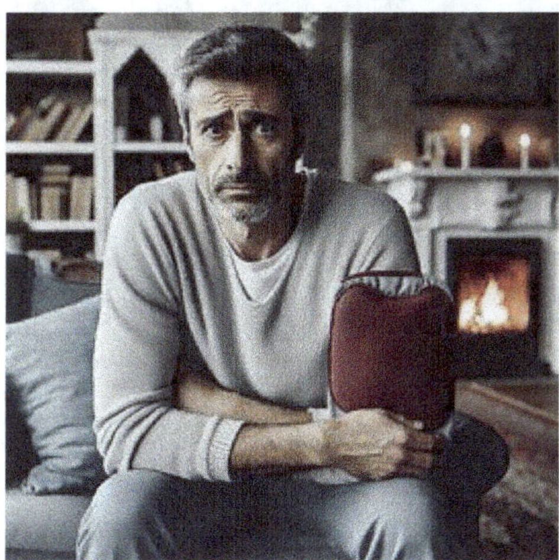

3. Fibromyalgia - Relieves pain, fatigue, and stiffness with gentle exercises and pain relief techniques.

4. Chronic obstructive pulmonary disease (COPD) - Breathing

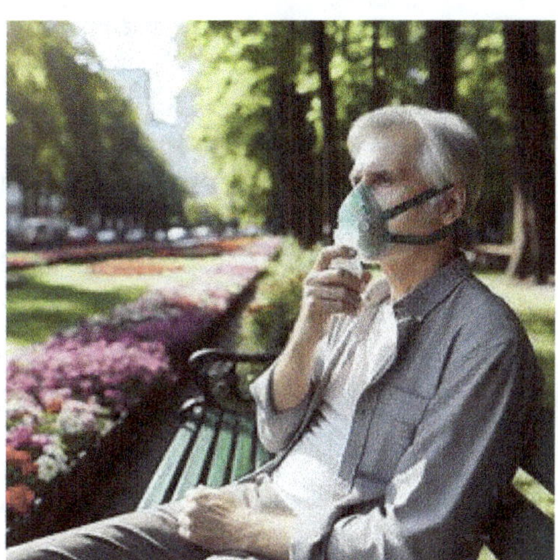

Regular physiotherapy sessions can also improve the quality of life by enhancing overall physical function and preventing further deterioration.

Overview of Physiotherapy :-

Physiotherapy, also known as physical therapy, is a healthcare profession that focuses on diagnosing, treating, and managing physical conditions that affect movement and function. The aim is to restore, maintain, and promote optimal physical functioning and quality of life. Physiotherapists use a variety of techniques, including exercises, manual therapy, modalities (e.g., heat, cold, electrical stimulation), and education to treat patients.

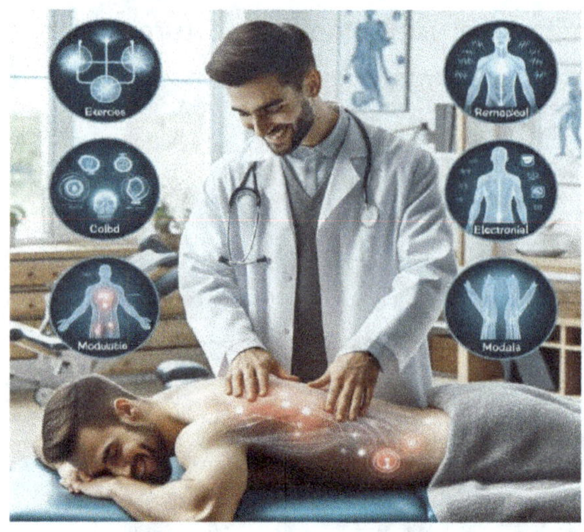

Key Aspects of Physiotherapy:

1. Assessment and Diagnosis:

Physiotherapists assess movement patterns, strength, flexibility, posture, and other physical aspects to diagnose conditions such as musculoskeletal disorders, neurological conditions, or respiratory issues.

2. Treatment Techniques:

• **Exercise Therapy:** Specific exercises are designed to improve strength, flexibility, balance, and coordination.

• **Manual Therapy:** Hands-on

techniques, such as massage and joint mobilization, to alleviate pain, reduce stiffness, and improve mobility.

• **Electrotherapy:** The use of electrical modalities like TENS (Transcutaneous Electrical Nerve Stimulation), ultrasound, or laser therapy for pain management and healing.

• **Posture and Ergonomics Training:** Education on proper posture and workplace ergonomics to prevent injuries.

3. Conditions Treated:

• **Musculoskeletal Issues:** Back pain, neck pain, joint pain, arthritis, and sports injuries.

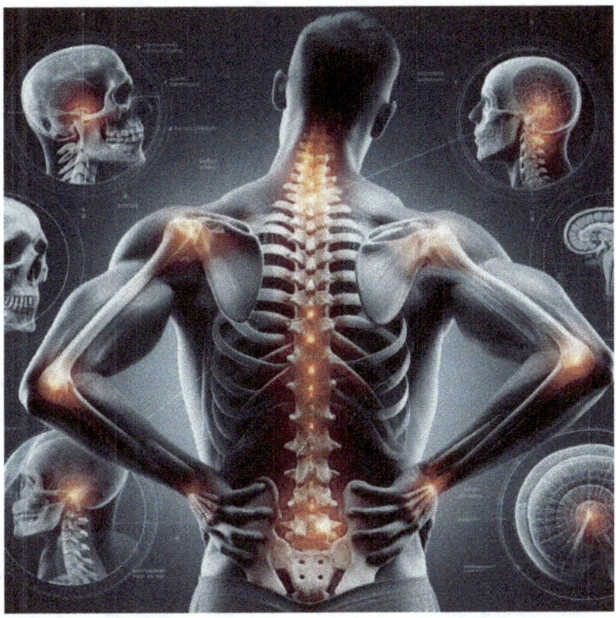

- **Neurological Disorders:** Stroke, Parkinson's disease, multiple sclerosis, and spinal cord injuries.

- **Cardiopulmonary Rehabilitation:** Treatment after heart surgery, lung conditions, or respiratory issues.

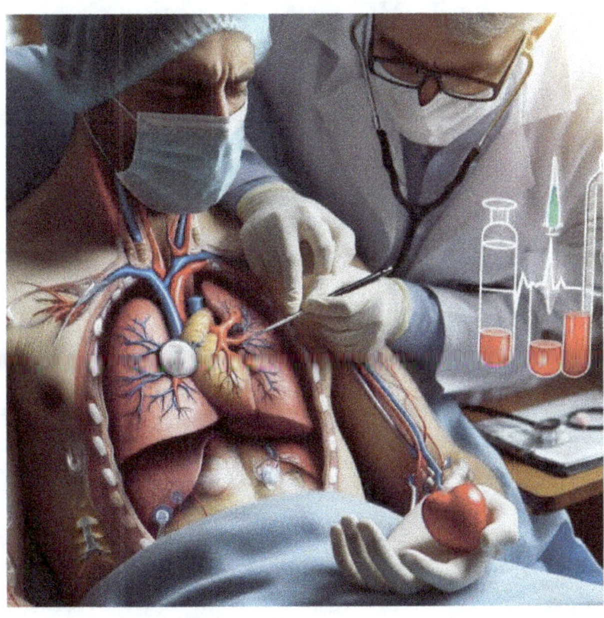

- **Pediatric and Geriatric Care:** Treatment for developmental issues in children or mobility concerns in older adults.

4. Goals of Physiotherapy:
- Reduce pain and inflammation
- Improve movement and mobility
- Prevent further injury or disability
- Enhance strength, endurance, and flexibility

• Educate patients for self-management of their condition

Physiotherapy can be provided in various settings such as hospitals, clinics, outpatient centers, sports teams, and even at home. It plays a crucial role in rehabilitation and promoting long-term health and well-being.

This structure would provide comprehensive coverage of physiotherapy in common people's lives. By expanding each section, focusing on easy-to-understand language, and using relatable examples, it can help readers understand the importance of physiotherapy and how it can be integrated into their lives for better health and well-being.